Case Study Workbook
Level 2

Printed in the U.S.A.

ISBN: 0=923369-57-0

Second Edition

101 West Buckingham Road, Richardson, TX 75081 1-800-443-7397

DISCLAIMER

Because each insurance company has its own processing and reimbursing policies, it is important that the coding student understand that the goals outlined herin are to learn coding according to the AMA's CPT-4 manual and to realze that the "rules" may change on the job which may or may not be in accordance with the AMA's CPT-4 book. It is critical that you check with each of your carriers to determine the applicability of the ideas outlined herein and determine each of their practices which could be unique to that carrier and which may not follow the guidelines set forth in **CPT** or **CP"Teach."**

Although the charts contained herein are original, the names of the patients and physicians have been changed to protect their anononimity.

ACKNOWLEDGMENTS

Some of the forms used in the OB/GYN section are part of the Hollister Maternal/Newborn Record System. Permission to reproduce this copyrighted material has been granted by the owner, Hollister Incorporated.

The **CP"Teach"** series includes some of the American Medical Association's **Physician's Current Procedural Terminology** descriptive terms, numeric identifying codes and modifiers for reporting medical services and procedures that were identified by the author, MedBooks, for inclusion in this book. **Physician's Current Procedural Terminology** is copyrighted (1966, 1970, 1973, 1977, 1981, 1983, 1984, 1985, 1986, 1987, 1988, 1989, 1990, 1991, 1992, 1993) by the American Medical Association. Any use of the **CPT** outside **CP"Teach"** should refer to **CPT** as it contains the most current listings of the descriptive terms, numeric services and procedures.

Suggestions on code additions or deletions in **CPT** should be directed to the American Medical Association at the following address:

Department of Coding and Nomenclature
CPT Publication
American Medical Association
515 North State Street
Chicago, Illinois 60610

DEDICATION

The Case Study Workbook is dedicated to the following physicians who unselfishly dedicated their time and energy in providing good, sound examples for use in this book.

Ben Darby, M.D.
Keller Griffith, M.D.
Thomas B. Hunter, M.D.
Irene Morin, M.D.
Norman Morin, M.D.
John Stubblefield, M.D.

I would also like to show my appreciation to my staff especially Jean Coats, Mary DeBauche, Anna Perez and Carol Vigna for their patience and understanding during the constant revisions. Of special importance is Becky Walters who has dedicated the better part of her heart, love and attitude into making this book what it is. My special thanks to all of you.

To Calla, my dear, dear daughter.
To her love and all the joy she brings to me.

Table of Contents

Case Study Workbook
Coding Questions

This book was formulated to give you the fullest sense of working in a physician's office. To accomplish this goal, each patient file is based on a real person (with all the names changed) and real doctor's records on each person. Below are questions that will ask you to code for a variety of services based on those patient files. All of the patients are arranged in alphabetical order in the next section and all the forms that you will need to code these services, such as HCFA 1500 and DocForms are also included. After completing the exercises in this workbook, you will have achieved the status of master coder. Good luck!

Evaluation and Management Services

Code each question for the date of service and the doctor indicated:

	Patient	Date of Service	Doctor	Specialty
1.	Walter Becca	March 2	Dr. S. Johns	DERM
2.	Albert Whitmore	October 31	Dr. Thomas	PS
3.	Albert Whitmore	November 6	Dr. Thomas	PS
4.	Albert Whitmore	December 11	Dr. Thomas	PS
5.	Evelyn Lindale	January 31	Dr. Thomas	PS
6.	James Edwards	October 2	Dr. Thomas	PS
7.	James Edwards	October 22	Dr. Thomas	PS
8.	Sandy Thompson	December 2	Dr. Thomas	PS
9.	Sandy Thompson	December 6	Dr. Thomas	PS
10.	Lawrence Brown	March 9	Dr. Thomas	PS
11.	April Hasty	October 21	Dr. Darby Bennata	OB/GYN
12.	April Hasty	November 15	Dr. Darby Bennata	OB/GYN
13.	April Hasty	November 17	Dr. Darby Bennata	OB/GYN
14.	April Hasty	December 9	Dr. Darby Bennata	OB/GYN

Evaluation and Management cont'd

Code each question for the date of service and the doctor indicated:

	Patient	Date of Service	Doctor	Specialty
15.	Bernice Saman	November 14	Dr. Darby Bennata	OB/GYN
16.	Bernice Saman	November 28	Dr. Darby Bennata	OB/GYN
17.	Beryl Hawthorne	November 21	Dr. Darby Bennata	OB/GYN
18.	Beryl Hawthorne	November 26	Dr. Darby Bennata	OB/GYN
19.	Beryl Hawthorne	February 10	Dr. Darby Bennata	OB/GYN
20.	Theresa Stacek	November 12	Dr. Darby Bennata	OB/GYN
21.	H.L. Stephens	February 6	Dr. M. Norman	ORTHO
22.	H.L. Stephens	February 12	Dr. M. Norman	ORTHO

Surgery

	Patient	Date of Service	Doctor	Specialty
23.	Walter Becca	February 16	Dr. S. Johns	DERM

How many follow-up days are considered included in the global fee period? Mark the global fee period in your chart.

24.	Albert Whitmore	October 30	Dr. Thomas	PS

How many follow-up days are considered included in the global fee period? Mark the global fee period in your chart.

25.	James Edwards	October 17	Dr. Thomas	PS

How many follow-up days are considered included in the global fee period? Mark the global fee period in your chart.

26.	Lawrence Brown	March 1	Dr. Thomas	PS

How many follow-up days are considered included in the global fee period? Mark the global fee period in your chart.

27.	April Hasty	November 15	Dr. Darby Bennata	OB/GYN

How many follow-up days are considered included in the global fee period? Mark the global fee period in your chart.

28.	Beryl Hawthorne	June 15	Dr. Darby Bennata	OB/GYN

How many follow-up days are considered included in the global fee period? Mark the global fee period in your chart.

29.	Theresa Stacek	November 7	Dr. Darby Bennata	OB/GYN

How many follow-up days are considered included in the global fee period? Mark the global fee period in your chart.

30.	Theresa Stacek	November 7	Dr. Perry Logan	OB/GYN

How many follow-up days are considered included in the global fee period? Mark the global fee period in your chart.

31.	Theresa Stacek	November 19	Dr. Perry Logan	OB/GYN

How many follow-up days are considered included in the global fee period? Mark the global fee period in your chart.

Radiology

Code each question for the date of service and the doctor indicated:

	Patient	Date of Service	Doctor	Specialty
32.	Meredith Dempsey	March 9	Dr. Sarah Mali	
33.	Albert Whitmore	October 30	Dr. R.R. John	
34.	Bernice Saman	May 7	Dr. Scott Davis	OB/GYN
35.	Bernice Saman	August 27	Dr. Scott Davis	OB/GYN
36.	Bernice Saman	November 13	Dr. Scott Davis	OB/GYN
37.	Beryl Hawthorne	September 19	Dr. Bryan James	OB/GYN
38.	Beryl Hawthorne	March 17	Dr. Bryan James	OB/GYN
39.	Theresa Stacek	October 26	Dr. Ray Davies	OB/GYN
40.	Theresa Stacek	March 18	Dr. Ray Enohose	OB/GYN
41.	Theresa Stacek	November 19	Dr. Bryan James	OB/GYN
42.	H.L. Stephens	February 6	Dr. M. Norman	ORTHO
43.	H.L. Stephens	February 12	Dr. R.N. Brown	ORTHO

Pathology

Code each question for the date of service and the doctor indicated:

	Patient	Date of Service	Doctor	Specialty
44.	Terry Spitz	March 11	Dr. Tom Rassler	OB/GYN
45.	April Hasty	November 15	Dr. G.L. Smith	OB/GYN
46.	Bernice Saman	July 12	Dr. Sam Stevens	OB/GYN
47.	Beryl Hawthorne	April 21	Dr. Renee Andrew	OB/GYN
48.	Theresa Stacek	April 15	Dr. Sam Stevens	OB/GYN

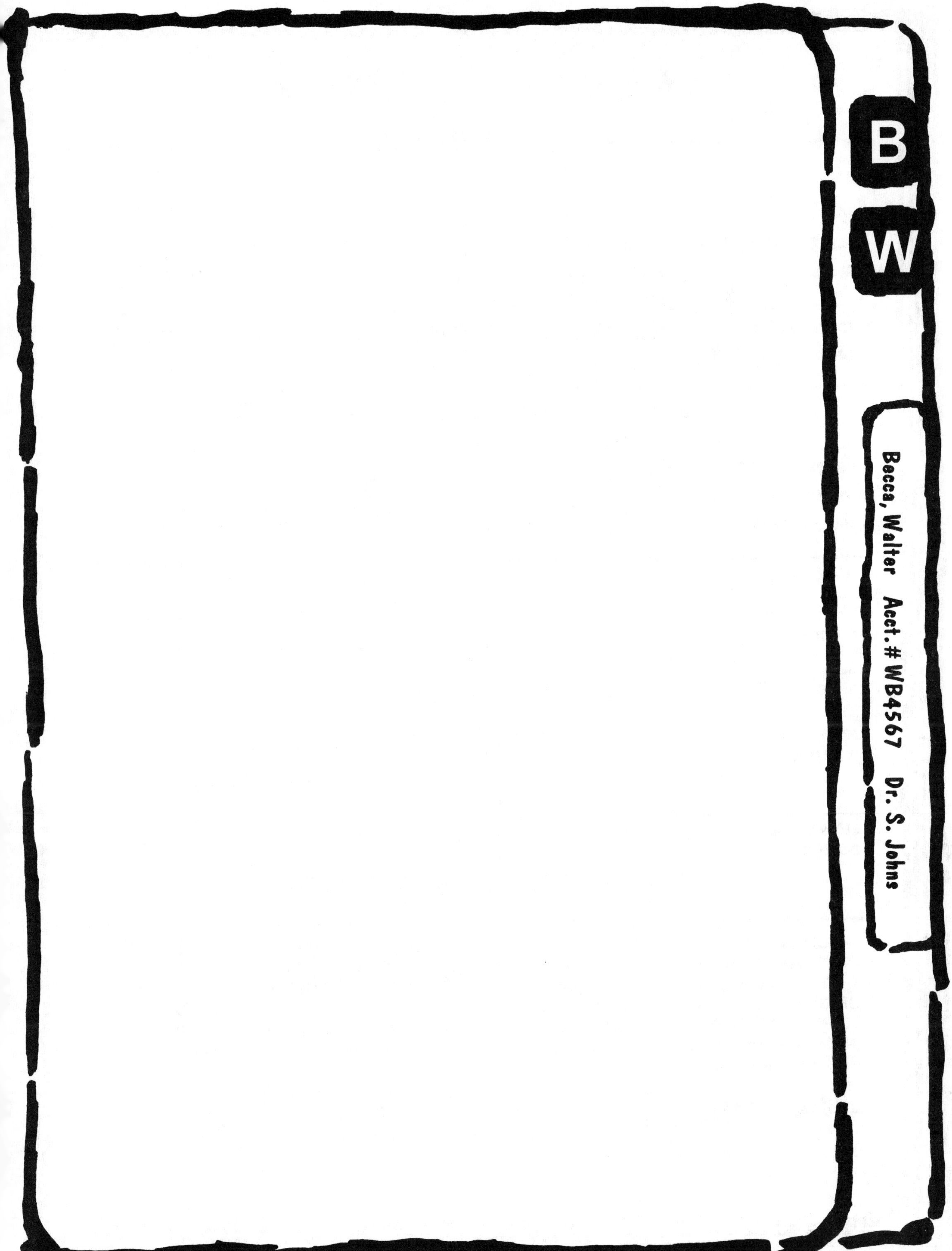

B
W
Becca, Walter Acct.# WB4567 Dr. S. Johns

Patient Information

PLEASE PRINT

PATIENT NAME Walter Becca AGE 37

ADDRESS 2456 Tulip Ave. BIRTHDATE 11-13

Paynesville, TX 77777 SEX M

SOCIAL SECURITY 111-22-3333 MARITAL STATUS M PHONE (713) 973-7397

EMPLOYER MedBooks PHONE (800) 443-7397

Please complete if patient is a minor or another party will be responsible for bill.

RESPONSIBLE PARTY Same RELATION ______

ADDRESS (IF DIFFERENT) ______

SOCIAL SECURITY ______ BIRTHDATE ______ PHONE ( ) ______

TYPE OF COVERAGE: MEDICARE MEDICAID (GROUP) SELF PAY OTHER

MEDICARE ______ PART A PART B

NAME ON CARD MEDICARE NUMBER

MEDICAID ______

NAME ON CARD MEDICAID NUMBER EFFECTIVE DATE

PRIMARY HEALTH INSURANCE BC/BS of Texas

COMPANY NAME ADDRESS

Walter Becca 7777WB88 WB555444

POLICY HOLDER POLICY NUMBER GROUP NUMBER

SECONDARY HEALTH INSURANCE ______

COMPANY NAME ADDRESS

POLICY HOLDER POLICY NUMBER GROUP NUMBER

I REQUEST THAT PAYMENT OF AUTHORIZED INSURANCE BENEFITS BE MADE EITHER TO ME OR ON MY BEHALF TO THE UNDERSIGNED PROVIDER FOR SERVICES FURNISHED ME BY THAT PHYSICIAN. I PERMIT A COPY OF THIS AUTHORIZATION TO BE USED IN PLACE OF MY ORIGINAL SIGNATURE AND AUTHORIZE ANY HOLDER OF MEDICAL INFORMATION ABOUT ME TO RELEASE TO THE HEALTH CARE FINANCING ADMINISTRATION OR ITS AGENTS ANY INFORMATION NEEDED TO DETERMINE THESE BENEFITS OR THE BENEFITS PAYABLE FOR RELATED SERVICES.

Walter Becca 2-16

PATIENT/GUARDIAN SIGNATURE DATE

Walter Becca

2/16 CC: Bleeding knot on forehead for last 2 mo

PI: Hx of sml lump developing on Ⓡ forehead 6 mo. ago but only in last 2 mo. has area bled. Hard, not irritating lesion.

PX: 0.8cm pearly ulcerated nodule c̄ a central crust located on Ⓡ forehead.

Imp: Basal cell epithelioma

Rx: ① Electrodessication + curettage c̄ biopsy under local Xylocaine

② Bactroban ointment to apply daily

③ Tylenol for pain

④ Return 2 wks.

3/2 Biopsy report reads as Basal cell. Forehead area healing fine

Disp: ① D/C Bactroban

② Return 1 mo.

B
L
Brown, Lawrence Acct. # LB5678 Dr. Thomas

Patient Information

PLEASE PRINT

PATIENT NAME Lawrence Brown AGE 75

ADDRESS 20 Sunnyvale Lane BIRTHDATE Jan 2

Pargueville Tx 77777 SEX M

SOCIAL SECURITY 000-11-2222 MARITAL STATUS S PHONE (713) 973-7357

EMPLOYER MedBooks PHONE (800) 443-7357

Please complete if patient is a minor or another party will be responsible for bill.

RESPONSIBLE PARTY ______ RELATION ______

ADDRESS (IF DIFFERENT) ______

SOCIAL SECURITY ______ BIRTHDATE ______ PHONE ( ) ______

TYPE OF COVERAGE: MEDICARE MEDICAID (GROUP) SELF PAY OTHER

MEDICARE ______ PART A PART B

NAME ON CARD MEDICARE NUMBER

MEDICAID ______

NAME ON CARD MEDICAID NUMBER EFFECTIVE DATE

PRIMARY HEALTH INSURANCE Humana

COMPANY NAME ADDRESS

Lawrence Brown 98754-765-4

POLICY HOLDER POLICY NUMBER GROUP NUMBER

SECONDARY HEALTH INSURANCE ______

COMPANY NAME ADDRESS

POLICY HOLDER POLICY NUMBER GROUP NUMBER

I REQUEST THAT PAYMENT OF AUTHORIZED INSURANCE BENEFITS BE MADE EITHER TO ME OR ON MY BEHALF TO THE UNDERSIGNED PROVIDER FOR SERVICES FURNISHED ME BY THAT PHYSICIAN. I PERMIT A COPY OF THIS AUTHORIZATION TO BE USED IN PLACE OF MY ORIGINAL SIGNATURE AND AUTHORIZE ANY HOLDER OF MEDICAL INFORMATION ABOUT ME TO RELEASE TO THE HEALTH CARE FINANCING ADMINISTRATION OR ITS AGENTS ANY INFORMATION NEEDED TO DETERMINE THESE BENEFITS OR THE BENEFITS PAYABLE FOR RELATED SERVICES.

Lawrence Brown Feb 10

PATIENT/GUARDIAN SIGNATURE DATE

2-10 L. Brown

75 y/o WM c̄ c/o growth ® cheek x n̂ i̇ year. PMH — HBP, emphysema RA, stroke PSH — appendectomy

Meds — theodur, tinoretic

allergies — ASA, codeine

PE: 3x2 cm ulcerative lesion c̄ rolled borders ® cheek.

Imp: Bc Ca

Recc: Excision c̄ FS + FC. Proc. explained in detail c̄ pt including risks, complications + alternative procedures. Pt wishes to schedule ASAP.

F.C. Thomas

3-9

i̇ wk post op. Incisions healing. SS applc'd. F/U c̄ Dr. Miller in 4 mos. Avoid sun exposure.

F.C. Thomas

Timothy Leary, M.D.
Family Practice Medicine
3232 Roustabout Lane
Payneville, TX 77777

February 27

Harold Thomas, M.D.
St. Patrick Tower Suite 232
Payneville, TX 77777

Dear Harold:

I would appreciate your taking a look at Mr. Lawrence Brown. As I am sure you know, Mr. Brown is the popular TV show host for "Let's Wheel and Deal." He appears to have had a growth on his right cheek (which he has had for the past three years). Mr. Brown enjoys playing golf and has greatly increased his time outside on the course since becoming such a TV star.

I am looking forward to your assistance in this case and will await your report.

Very truly yours,

Timothy Leary, M.D.

TL/br

REPORT OF OPERATION

St. Patrick Hospital
Payneville, Texas 77777

		Case #	21		
Name	Lawrence Brown	Date	March 1	Room #	Outpatient
Surgeon	Dr. Thomas	Assistant			
Anesthetist		Started		Ended	

Preoperative Diagnosis: Basal cell carcinoma right cheek

Postoperative Diagnosis: Same

Operation: Excision of basal cell carcinoma right cheek with bilateral advancement flaps for wound closure.

INDICATIONS FOR PROCEDURE:
This 75-year-old white male was referred to my office for evaluation of an ulcerative growth on his right cheek which had been present for several years. Clinically the lesion had a central ulceration with rolled borders and measured approximately 4.5 x 2.5 cm. It appeared to be a basal cell carcinoma. There were no cervical nodes palpable on physical exam.

PROCEDURE IN DETAIL:
The patient was placed on the operating room table in the supine position and the head and neck were prepared and draped in the sterile fashion. A skin marker was used to outline a planned excision which measured 7 x 3 cm. The lesion was excised after infiltrating with local anesthesia. Bleeding was controlled with the electrocautery unit. The wound was marked in the 12 o'clock position and sent for frozen section. Path report returned with conclusion of basal cell carcinoma which was completely excised. The medial portion of the cheek skin was then elevated under direct vision using Metzenbaum scissors. The lateral preauricular skin was also elevated in a similar fashion. The elevation was continued in both directions medially and laterally for approximately 4 cm taking care to stay in the subcutaneous unit. The flaps were advanced and inset using interrupted buried 5-0 Vicryl followed by interrupted 5-0 nylon on the skin. The wound was dressed with Polysporin ointment. The patient tolerated the procedure well.

DR. H. Thomas/md
CC
DICT: March 1
TRAN: March 2

D

M

Dempsy, Meredith Acct. # MD8901 Dr. R. Jonson

Patient Information

PLEASE PRINT

PATIENT NAME Meredith Dempsy AGE 36
ADDRESS 315 Alamo St. BIRTHDATE 1-5
Payneville TX 77777 SEX F
SOCIAL SECURITY 523-42-8193 MARITAL STATUS M PHONE (713) 973-7391
EMPLOYER MedBooks PHONE (800) 443-7397

Please complete if patient is a minor or another party will be responsible for bill.

RESPONSIBLE PARTY ______ RELATION ______
ADDRESS (IF DIFFERENT) ______
SOCIAL SECURITY ______ BIRTHDATE ______ PHONE ( ) ______

TYPE OF COVERAGE: MEDICARE MEDICAID GROUP SELF PAY OTHER (circled)

MEDICARE ______ PART A PART B
NAME ON CARD MEDICARE NUMBER

MEDICAID ______
NAME ON CARD MEDICAID NUMBER EFFECTIVE DATE

PRIMARY HEALTH INSURANCE
Equitable (COMPANY NAME) P.O. Box 65000 Dallas TX (ADDRESS)
Meredith Dempsy (POLICY HOLDER) MD523-42-8193 (POLICY NUMBER) GROUP NUMBER

SECONDARY HEALTH INSURANCE ______
COMPANY NAME ADDRESS
POLICY HOLDER POLICY NUMBER GROUP NUMBER

I REQUEST THAT PAYMENT OF AUTHORIZED INSURANCE BENEFITS BE MADE EITHER TO ME OR ON MY BEHALF TO THE UNDERSIGNED PROVIDER FOR SERVICES FURNISHED ME BY THAT PHYSICIAN. I PERMIT A COPY OF THIS AUTHORIZATION TO BE USED IN PLACE OF MY ORIGINAL SIGNATURE AND AUTHORIZE ANY HOLDER OF MEDICAL INFORMATION ABOUT ME TO RELEASE TO THE HEALTH CARE FINANCING ADMINISTRATION OR ITS AGENTS ANY INFORMATION NEEDED TO DETERMINE THESE BENEFITS OR THE BENEFITS PAYABLE FOR RELATED SERVICES.

Mrs. Meredith Dempsy 3-9
PATIENT/GUARDIAN SIGNATURE DATE

Sarah Mali, M.D., P.A.
Diagnostic Ultrasound and Mammography
St. Patrick Tower, Suite 608
Payneville, TX 77777

TO DR:	*Jonson*	OB:		
REPORT ON:	*Dempsy, Meredith*	SOC SEC #:	*523-42-8193*	
DATE OF EXAM:	*March 9*	AGE:	*36 YRS*	*PAGE 1 OF 3*

IMPRESSION

16.3 week single viable intrauterine pregnancy.
No gross fetal abnormalities are identified on this sonogram.
The fetal growth appears to be in the normal range.

SM/sb

Sarah Mali, M.D.

FETAL NUMBER AND POSITION:

A single fetus is noted in complete breech presentation.

PLACENTA:

The placenta appears to be on the left side, anterior and posterior, in grade 0, LOW LYING, with no gross evidence of placenta previa on examination with an empty and partially full bladder. The position of the placenta is expected to improve in later periods of gestation. Negative for evidence of gross abruption of the placenta.

AMNIOTIC FLUID:

The amniotic fluid appears to be normal in quantity.

UMBILICAL CORD:

Three vessel umbilical cord is seen.

DOPPLER AND COLOR FLOW EXAMINATION:

Brief pulsed doppler and color flow examination reveals the umbilical arterial velocity waveform to be in the normal range.

MATERNAL CERVIX:

The maternal cervix appears to be normal in size with no evidence of dilatation of the lower uterine segment.

FETAL CNS:

The fetal head, normal sized lateral ventricles, choroid plexus, thalami, cerebral peduncles, symmetrical intracranial structures, cerebellum are identified.

The cervical, thoracic, lumbar and sacral spine were scanned from multiple projections, appearing to be unremarkable on sonogram.

FETAL FACE:

The fetal face, both orbits, bony nostrils, mandible, mouth are present. Please note that the fetal face is difficult to examine due to early fetal age.

FETAL CARDIOVASCULAR SYSTEM:

Cardiac activity is noted with regular cardiac rhythm. The ventricular chambers appear to be equal in size with good ventricular wall motions. The four chambers of the heart, mitral tricuspid valves, interventricular septum, aortic root, pulmonary trunk are seen. Please note the limitations of sonography in the evaluation of the fetal heart and great vessels particularly due to early age.

FETAL CHEST AND LUNGS:

The fetal chest, lungs, diaphragm are seen.

FETAL GI:

The fetal right kidney, left kidney, normal size bladder are seen. Please note the limitations of sonography to evaluate the fetal kidneys and bladder particularly due to early age.

FETAL SKELETAL SYSTEM:

The fetal right arm, left arm, right leg, left leg are seen. Both hands and feet are noted. The long bones on both sides are visualized and appear to be unremarkable in length and ossification, with no evidence of gross deformities or abnormal curvatures of the bones.

FETAL MOVEMENTS:

The movements of the fetal head, body and extremities are seen.

FETAL SEX:

The fetus appears to be female.
The patient does not wish to know the sex of the baby.

MATERNAL RIGHT AND LEFT OVARY AND PELVIS:

Negative for gross adnexal mass.

OTHER COMMENTS:

High maternal age is noted and the fetus carefully scanned. Please note the limitations of sonography in the evaluation of the fetus, particularly due to early fetal age, and that a negative sonogram does not guarantee a perfect baby.

PAGE 2 OF 3
PT. NAME DEMPSY, MEREDITH DR. Jonson March 9

NAME:	*DEMPSY, MEREDITH*	REF PHYSICIAN:	*DR. Jonson*
AGE:	*36*	EXAM DATE:	*3/9*

FETAL MEASUREMENTS:		GESTATIONAL AGE:			
RANGE:					
BPD(CM)	3.40	GA BY BPD	(WKS)	16.0	15.0-17.0
HC(CM)	12.09	GA BY HC	(WKS)	16.3	15.3-17.3
AC(CM)	10.36	GA BY AC	(WKS)	16.5	15.5-17.5
FEMUR(CM)	2.0	GA BY FL	(WKS)	16.3	15.3-17.3
OOD(CM)	2.5	GA BY OD	(WKS)	16.0	15.0-17.0
LMP	11/13/94	GA BY LMP	(WKS)	16.6	

LAT VENT	0.6	H/A RATIO	1.17	NORMAL 1.05-1.39
OFD(CM)	4.3	CEPHALIC INDEX	79.1	
IOD(CM)	1.0	FETAL HEART RATE	149.0	
ABD DIAM	3.3	TIBIA(CM)	1.7	
FL/BPD	0.59	HUMERUS(CM)	2.0	
FL/HC	0.17	ULNA(CM)	1.8	
FL/AC	0.19	RADIUS(CM)	1.6	
CAL EPI		TALAR EPI		
DFE		PTE		

(FL/AC)x100	(Normal 22.3 +/- 2.4)	19.30
(TIBIA/AC)x100	(Normal 19.3 +/- 2.2)	16.41
(FL+TIBIA/AC)x100	(Normal 41.6 +/- 4.2)	35.71

TRANSVERSE CEREBELLAR DIAMETER (MM)

FETAL BIOPHYSICAL PROFILE: WITHIN NORMAL LIMITS

AVERAGE FETAL AGE (WKS): 16.3 SELECTED AGE (WKS)

ESTD DATE OF DELIVERY BY LMP: 08/20
ESTD DATE OF DELIVERY BY SCAN: 08/22

(PLEASE NOTE THAT THE ESTIMATED WEIGHT BY SONOGRAM MAY VARY BY MORE THAN 20 PERCENT FROM THE ACTUAL FETAL BODY WEIGHT)

ESTD FETAL WEIGHT	GMS	LBS	AND OZ
BY (BPD,AC)	169.9	0	6.0
BY (BPD,HC,AC,FL)	169.1	0	6.0
AVERAGE FETAL WT	169.5	0	6.0

The estimated sonographic fetal age is the menstrual age of the fetus.

PAGE 3 OF 3

SARAH MALI, M.D.

D

M

E
J
Edwards, James Acct.# JE4234 Dr. Thomas

Patient Information

PLEASE PRINT

PATIENT NAME JAMES EDWARDS AGE 44

ADDRESS 41 Plaza Square BIRTHDATE 6/2

Payneville, Tx 77777 SEX M

SOCIAL SECURITY 666-44-0000 MARITAL STATUS M PHONE (713) 973-7397

EMPLOYER Med Books PHONE (800) 443-7397

Please complete if patient is a minor or another party will be responsible for bill.

RESPONSIBLE PARTY ______ RELATION ______

ADDRESS (IF DIFFERENT) ______

SOCIAL SECURITY ______ BIRTHDATE ______ PHONE ( ) ______

TYPE OF COVERAGE: MEDICARE MEDICAID GROUP SELF PAY (OTHER)

MEDICARE ______ PART A PART B

NAME ON CARD MEDICARE NUMBER

MEDICAID ______

NAME ON CARD MEDICAID NUMBER EFFECTIVE DATE

PRIMARY HEALTH INSURANCE Travelers

COMPANY NAME ADDRESS

James Edwards 875-3427-990

POLICY HOLDER POLICY NUMBER GROUP NUMBER

SECONDARY HEALTH INSURANCE ______

COMPANY NAME ADDRESS

POLICY HOLDER POLICY NUMBER GROUP NUMBER

I REQUEST THAT PAYMENT OF AUTHORIZED INSURANCE BENEFITS BE MADE EITHER TO ME OR ON MY BEHALF TO THE UNDERSIGNED PROVIDER FOR SERVICES FURNISHED ME BY THAT PHYSICIAN. I PERMIT A COPY OF THIS AUTHORIZATION TO BE USED IN PLACE OF MY ORIGINAL SIGNATURE AND AUTHORIZE ANY HOLDER OF MEDICAL INFORMATION ABOUT ME TO RELEASE TO THE HEALTH CARE FINANCING ADMINISTRATION OR ITS AGENTS ANY INFORMATION NEEDED TO DETERMINE THESE BENEFITS OR THE BENEFITS PAYABLE FOR RELATED SERVICES.

James Edwards 10-2

PATIENT/GUARDIAN SIGNATURE DATE

10-2 James Edwards

44 y/o WM c̄ c/o recent change in color + size of several moles on his face. Pt is concerned about the possibility of malignancy and would like the moles removed for bx. PMH - Ø.

PE:

Ⓡ eyelid — 5×5 mm raised, tan lesion
Ⓡ cheek — 1×1 cm " " "
nose — 5×5 mm " " "
Ⓛ cheek — 1×1 cm " " "
neck — 5×5 mm " dark tan lesion

Imp — intradermal nevi X5 on face
R/O melanoma

Recc — Excisional bx X5. Procedure explained in detail c̄ pt. including risks, complications + alternate procedures. Pt understands he will have scarring. Pt wishes to schedule ASAP.

10-22 J. Edwards.

1 wk post-op. Incisions healing well.
SS out + steri-strips applied. RTC 1 mo.

REPORT OF OPERATION

St. Patrick Hospital
Payneville, Texas 77777

		Case #:	JE4234		
Name:	James Edwards	**Date:**	10-17	**Room #:**	
Surgeon:	H. Thomas	**Assistant:**	None		
Anesthetist:		**Started:**		**Ended:**	

Preoperative Diagnosis: Multiple nevi to face and neck
R/O Melanoma

Postoperative Diagnosis: same

Operation: Excision of nevi from the face and neck

Anesthesia: 1% Xylocaine with Epinephrine and Sodium Bicarbonate

INDICATIONS: Patient was referred to my office by his primary care physician for evaluation of several nevi on the face which had increased in size over the past several months. On physical examination the patient had multiple nevi on the face and neck most of which appeared to be benign intradermal nevi.

PROCEDURE: The patient was placed on the OR table in the supine position and the head/neck area was prepped and draped in a sterile fashion. The following nevi were marked for removal and individual biopsy. 1. right cheek 1x1 cm; 2. nose 5x5 mm; 3. left cheek 1x1 cm; 4. neck 5x5 mm; 5. right eyelid 5x5 mm. Each of these areas was infiltrated with a local anesthesia and a #15 blade was used to circumferentially excise all of the lesion. Bleeding was controlled with the electrocautery unit; all wounds were closed using simple sutures with interrupted 5-0 nylon except for the right eyelid lesion which was closed with interrupted 6-0 nylon. Neosporin ointment and steri-strips were applied to all suture lines. The patient tolerated the procedure well.

HT/md
CC:
DICT: Oct 17
TRAN: Oct 17

E

J

H
A
Hasty, April Acct.# AH8502 Dr. Bennata

Patient Information

PLEASE PRINT

PATIENT NAME APRIL HASTY AGE 64
ADDRESS RT 2 BOX 644 BIRTHDATE 2/18
PAYNEVILLE, TX 77777 SEX F
SOCIAL SECURITY 212-33-4545 MARITAL STATUS M PHONE (713) 973-7397
EMPLOYER ______ PHONE ( ) ______

Please complete if patient is a minor or another party will be responsible for bill.

RESPONSIBLE PARTY ______ RELATION ______
ADDRESS (IF DIFFERENT) ______
SOCIAL SECURITY ______ BIRTHDATE ______ PHONE ( ) ______

TYPE OF COVERAGE: MEDICARE MEDICAID (GROUP) SELF PAY OTHER

MEDICARE ______ PART A PART B
NAME ON CARD MEDICARE NUMBER

MEDICAID ______
NAME ON CARD MEDICAID NUMBER EFFECTIVE DATE

PRIMARY HEALTH INSURANCE EQUITABLE DALLAS, TX
COMPANY NAME ADDRESS
CHARLES HASTY 6789123
POLICY HOLDER POLICY NUMBER GROUP NUMBER

SECONDARY HEALTH INSURANCE ______
COMPANY NAME ADDRESS
______
POLICY HOLDER POLICY NUMBER GROUP NUMBER

I REQUEST THAT PAYMENT OF AUTHORIZED INSURANCE BENEFITS BE MADE EITHER TO ME OR ON MY BEHALF TO THE UNDERSIGNED PROVIDER FOR SERVICES FURNISHED ME BY THAT PHYSICIAN. I PERMIT A COPY OF THIS AUTHORIZATION TO BE USED IN PLACE OF MY ORIGINAL SIGNATURE AND AUTHORIZE ANY HOLDER OF MEDICAL INFORMATION ABOUT ME TO RELEASE TO THE HEALTH CARE FINANCING ADMINISTRATION OR ITS AGENTS ANY INFORMATION NEEDED TO DETERMINE THESE BENEFITS OR THE BENEFITS PAYABLE FOR RELATED SERVICES.

April Hasty 10/21
PATIENT/GUARDIAN SIGNATURE DATE

April Hasty

10/21 age 64
c/o "bladder falling"
Physical & pap · 2 wks ago BP 170/80
Pregnancies III Children III D&C 1983
Bladder fallen for several mos. Extends
out of opening of vagina.
2° cystocele, 2° uterine prolapse
Tx Plan · meds vs. benefit of total ab.
hysterectomy. Bladder suspension anterior
Repair discussed in detail - failure of
procedure stressed.

11/23 Two P.O. TAH BSO appendectomy A+P
repair TAH. B.P 154/92. ↑ stitch removed
no other complaints. Abd. healing fine.
Return 2 wks.

12/5 3 wks. P.O. TAH B.P. 142/86 no complaints
cervix healing cuff intact. Uterus - no masses
Abd. - no masses. - Return 3 wks.

12/27 5 wks P.O. TAH B.P. 164/94 no vasometer
symptoms. Cuff intact. no masses found in
uterus or abdomen. no swelling present in
abdomen. Return 6 mos.

WEST
CAL-CAM
HOSPITAL

HISTORY SHEET

NAME: Hasty, April DATE: 11-15 ROOM NO.:
ATTENDING PHYSICIAN: Darby, Bennata
CHIEF COMPLAINT: Pelvic dragging sensation

PRESENT ILLNESS:

The patient is a 64 year old G-III P-III who has a history of symptomatic uterine descensus and symptomatic cystocele who is admitted for transabdominal hysterectomy bilateral salpingo-oophorectomy and vaginal vault suspension. The patient also has a history of symptomatic rectocele.

PAST HISTORY:

SURGICAL: D&C 1983
MEDICAL: The patient has a history of hypothyroidism.
ALLERGIES: None.
CHILDHOOD: Usual illnesses.
FAMILY HISTORY: Positive for diabetes mellitus.
SOCIAL HISTORY: The patient denies use of ethanol or tobacco.

ROS:

GENERAL: No chills, fever, night sweats.
HEENT: No tinnitus, diplopia, epistaxis.
CARDIORESPIRATORY: Denies chest pain, PND or DOE.
GI: No nausea, vomiting, diarrhea, or melena.
GU: See present illness.
NM: Noncontributory.

WEST
CAL-CAM
HOSPITAL

PHYSICAL EXAMINATION

NAME: Hasty, April DATE: 11-15 ROOM NO.:
ATTENDING PHYSICIAN: Darby Bennata, M.D.

VITAL SIGNS: TEMP: 99.7 PULSE 64 RESP: 20 BP: 150/84

GENERAL: The patient is alert and oriented to time and place, and in no apparent distress.

SKIN: Good turgor, texture and coloration.

HEENT: Normocephalic, PERRLA, EOM's intact, fundi benign, tympanic membranes, external ear canals clear bilaterally.

NECK: Supple, full range of motion. No lymphadenopathy or thyromegaly. Pharynx within normal limits, no bruits or JVD noted.

CHEST: Clear to auscultation and percussion, no rales, rubs or rhonchi. Good symmetry with good inspiratory effort, no gross deformity.

HEART: Regular rhythm without murmur or gallop. S1 and S2 within normal limits. PMI at the left intercostal space and in the midclavicular line.

ABDOMEN: Soft, bowel sounds normal active, no CVA, rebound, or tenderness is noted.

PELVIC EXAM: External genitalia, normal female escutcheon. BUS, negative. Vagina, normal mucosa with a mild +1 cystocele and +2 rectocele present. The cervix descends to a +2 station. Uterus is upper limits of normal in size and slightly tender. Adnexal regions are tender bilaterally with no definite masses.

EXTREMITIES: No cyanosis, clubbing, or edema. Full range of motion in all joints. Distal pulses are equal.

NEUROLOGICAL: Cranial nerves 2 through 12 are grossly intact. Deep tendon reflexes are 2+ out 3+ and bilaterally equal. No abnormal reflexes are elicited.

IMPRESSION: SYMPTOMATIC UTERINE DESCENDUS
SYMPTOMATIC CYSTOCELE AND RECTOCELE

REPORT OF OPERATION

WEST
CAL-CAM
HOSPITAL

NAME: Hasty, April
DATE OF PROCEDURE: 11-15
PREOPERATIVE DIAGNOSIS: Symptomatic Uterine Descendus
Symptomatic Cystocele
POSTOPERATIVE DIAGNOSIS: Same
OPERATION PERFORMED: Transabdominal hysterectomy
Bilateral Salpingo-Oophorectomy
Appendectomy
Posterior Colporrhaphy

After discussing the diagnosis and proposed procedure along with the risks and complications informed consent was obtained. Routine premedications were given. The patient was brought to the Operating Room and prepped and draped in the routine fashion. Abdominal and vaginal preparation consisted of Betadine scrub sponges followed by Betadine solution swabs. General anesthesia was administered by the nurse anesthetist.

Pfannenstiel incision was made and sharp dissection was carried through the subcutaneous tissue to the fascia which was identified and incised. Blunt and sharp dissection was carried down to the peritoneum which was identified and incised. Inspection of the pelvic viscera revealed the presence of a uterus which is extremely mobile on its ligamentous supports. The uterus was noted to be studded with multiple uterine leiomyomata. The ovaries are noted to be atrophic bilaterally. The right round ligament was grasped with an Ochsner clamp, suture ligated times one using a #1 chromic atraumatic suture. Dissection was then carried down the anterior leaf of the broad ligament to the vesicouterine fold. A finger was placed bluntly through the quadrangular avascular space and a #1 chromic free hand ligature was used to ligate the right infundibulopelvic ligament. This was followed by clamping and transection followed by suture ligation times one using a #1 chromic atraumatic suture. Good hemostasis ensued. The exact same procedure was carried out on the left with good resulting hemostasis.

The uterine arteries were then bilaterally doubly Heaney clamped, cut, and suture ligated times two using #1 chromic atraumatic sutures. Good hemostasis ensued. Bilateral serial Ochsner clamping against the cervix of the cardinal ligaments was then carried out with each successive pedicle being ligated time one using #1 chromic atraumatic sutures. Good hemostasis ensued. At the level of the uterosacral ligaments a curved Heaney clamp was used to grasp the uterosacral ligament which was then transected. Each ligament was then suture ligated times two using #1 chromic atraumatic sutures. The vaginal cavity was entered laterally and the specimen was excised from the field and submitted to the pathologist for evaluation. Modified Aldridge angle sutures were placed bilaterally and the anterior and posterior vaginal cuff were closed individually using #1 chromic running and locking sutures. The cuff was then closed using #1 chromic figure of eight sutures. The pelvic cavity was lavaged with warm normal saline and inspection of the pelvic sidewalls, cuff, and posterior bladder revealed good hemostasis. Reperitonealization was then carried out using 2-0 chromic running sutures. The appendix was grasped by Babcock clamps and elevated into the operative field.

The mesoappendix was serially clamped, cut and ligated using 3-0 black silk sutures. At the base of the appendix 3-0 black silk purse-string was placed around the base. The appendix was then transected and submitted to the pathologist for evaluation. The appendiceal stump was then inverted into the purse-string suture which was then secured. Good hemostasis was noted. Lap, sponge and needle count were noted to be correct and reinspection revealed good hemostasis. The peritoneum was closed using 0 chromic running sutures. Fascial closure was carried out using 2-0 plain interrupted sutures and the skin was closed with 3-0 Vicryl subcuticular sutures. The patient's wound was dressed in a sterile fashion and lap, sponge, and needle count were noted to be correct a second time.

The patient was taken to the Recovery Room with stable vital signs and draining clear urine.

REPORT OF OPERATION

WEST
CAL-CAM
HOSPITAL

NAME:
PAGE 2

Hasty, April

continued...

ADDENDUM:

The posterior fourchette was draped in a routine fashion and Allis clamps were used to grasp the mucocutaneous junction of the vagina at 5 o'clock and 7 o'clock respectively. An Allis clamp was then placed in the vaginal vault in the midline approximately 2 cm from the vaginal cuff. A triangular section of vaginal mucosa was then reflected and excised. Three #1 chromic atraumatic plication sutures were placed in the posterior vaginal fascia and secured. Good hemostasis ensued and the subcutaneous layer was closed using 2-0 chromic interrupted sutures. Vaginal mucosa closure was carried out using 2-0 chromic interrupted sutures. Good hemostasis ensued.

A Cooper ligament suspension of the vaginal cuff was carried out by using a 0 Novafil interrupted suture to secure the right vaginal fornix to the posterior Cooper ligament. This was carried out x 2.

Estimated blood loss: 300 cc

Darby Bennata, M.D.
dd: 11-15
dt: 11-16
mct

WEST
CAL-CAM
HOSPITAL

PATHOLOGY REPORT

NAME: Hasty, April
DATE OF PROCEDURE: 11-15
PREOPERATIVE DIAGNOSIS: Symptomatic Cystocele; Symptomatic Uterine Descensus.

POSTOPERATIVE DIAGNOSIS: Same.
BRIEF CLINICAL HISTORY: None given
SPECIMEN:
A. Uterus, cervix, bilateral fallopian tubes and ovaries.
B. Appendix.
C. Posterior repair tissue.

GROSS:
A. Uterus, cervix, bilateral fallopian tubes and ovaries 100 grams measuring 9 x 5 x 4 cm with multiple leiomyomas present in the mucosal area 1.3 cm and also in the mucosa and submucosal and intermural area varying from 0.3 to 0.8 cm. There is an endocervical polyp 2 cm. Cervix is congested. Representative sections submitted. Bilateral fallopian tubes are unremarkable except for peritubal cyst on the left side. The ovaries are unremarkable. The right ovary is 3 x 1 x 0.5 and the left ovary is 2 x 1 x 0.6 cm. The ovaries are atrophic.
B. Appendix 6 x 0.4 cm.
C. Posterior repair tissue consists of two pieces of vaginal mucosa. Representative sections submitted.

MICROSCOPIC:
A. The section of the endometrium shows thin endometrium with scanty, round and tubular proliferative type glands and stroma. The cervix shows hyperkeratosis, focal parakeratosis, multiple cystic endocervical glands. A large endocervical polyp shows the tip with extensive squamous metaplasia. Endometrial polyp shows cystic hyperplasia. In some of the leiomyomas there is hyalinized changes in the stroma. Ovaries are atrophic with corpora albecans and also small peritubal cyst.
B. Appendix shows intact wall without evidence of active inflammatory changes.
C. Vaginal mucosa is congested with no atypia.

DIAGNOSIS: Uterus, cervix, bilateral fallopian tubes and ovaries:
MULTIPLE LEIOMYOMAS.
MUCOSAL, SUBMUCOSAL, AND INTERMURAL
ENDOMETRIAL POLYP WITH CYSTIC HYPERPLASIA.
CERVICAL POLYP WITH SQUAMOUS METAPLASIA.
CYSTIC ENDOCERVICAL GLANDS.
BILATERAL FALLOPIAN TUBES.
ONE FALLOPIAN TUBE WITH PERITUBAL CYST.
OVARIES, ATROPHIC.
Vermiform appendix.
Posterior vaginal tissue.

G.L. Smith, M.D.
GLS/nk

DISCHARGE SUMMARY

WEST
CAL-CAM
HOSPITAL

NAME: Hasty, April ADMIT DATE: 11-15 DISCHARGE DATE: 11-17
ATTENDING PHYSICIAN: Darby Bennata, M.D.

BRIEF HISTORY: The patient is a 64 year old G-8 P-3 with a history of symptomatic uterine descensus and symptomatic cystocele and rectocele admitted for repair.

PERTINENT PHYSICAL FINDINGS: Physical findings include a +1 cystocele, +2 rectocele, and uterine descensus. The uterus is upper limits of normal in size.

PERTINENT LABORATORY FINDINGS: Admission hematocrit 43%. White blood cell count 5,000. Blood type A+.

HOSPITAL COURSE:
The patient was admitted and after preoperative evaluation underwent TAH BSO appendectomy posterior repair with Cooper ligament suspension of the vaginal vault. By the first postoperative day, the patient was tolerating a diet and ambulating without assistance. By the second postoperative day, the patient was tolerating a diet and passing flatus and was discharged. She was instructed to return to the office on 11-23 and given a prescription for Duricef 500 q 12 hours x 10 days, Percoset 1 or 2 PO q 4 hours prn pain. The patient was instructed to notify me for any temperature of 100 or above, increasing abdominal or pelvic pain, vaginal bleeding, or other problems. She was instructed in hydrogen peroxide wound care and a regular diet.

FINAL DIAGNOSIS:
SYMPTOMATIC UTERINE DESCENSUS
SYMPTOMATIC CYSTOCELE
MULTIPLE UTERINE LEIOMYOMAS
ENDOMETRIAL POLYP WITH CYSTIC HYPERPLASIA
SQUAMOUS METOPLASIA, CERVICAL POLYP

OPERATIVE PROCEDURES:
TRANSABDOMINAL HYSTERECTOMY
BILATERAL SALPINGO-OOPHORECTOMY
APPENDECTOMY
POSTERIOR COLPORRHAPHY
COOPER LIGAMENT SUSPENSION OF THE VAGINAL VAULT

Darby Bennata, M.D.
dd: 11-15
dt: 11-16
mc

H
B
Hawthorne, Beryl Acct.# BH8501 Dr. Bennata

Patient Information

PLEASE PRINT

PATIENT NAME Beryl Hawthorne AGE 18

ADDRESS 1256 S. Yale Boulevard BIRTHDATE 12/23

Payneville, Texas SEX F

SOCIAL SECURITY 333-44-2222 MARITAL STATUS S PHONE (713) 555-7042

EMPLOYER MedBooks PHONE (800) 443-7397

Please complete if patient is a minor or another party will be responsible for bill.

RESPONSIBLE PARTY ______ RELATION ______

ADDRESS (IF DIFFERENT) ______

SOCIAL SECURITY ______ BIRTHDATE ______ PHONE ( ) ______

TYPE OF COVERAGE: MEDICARE MEDICAID (GROUP) SELF PAY OTHER

MEDICARE ______ PART A PART B

NAME ON CARD MEDICARE NUMBER

MEDICAID ______

NAME ON CARD MEDICAID NUMBER EFFECTIVE DATE

PRIMARY HEALTH INSURANCE

Equitable (COMPANY NAME) Dallas, Texas (ADDRESS)

Beryl Hawthorne (POLICY HOLDER) 213BH714 (POLICY NUMBER) GROUP NUMBER

SECONDARY HEALTH INSURANCE

COMPANY NAME ADDRESS

POLICY HOLDER POLICY NUMBER GROUP NUMBER

I REQUEST THAT PAYMENT OF AUTHORIZED INSURANCE BENEFITS BE MADE EITHER TO ME OR ON MY BEHALF TO THE UNDERSIGNED PROVIDER FOR SERVICES FURNISHED ME BY THAT PHYSICIAN. I PERMIT A COPY OF THIS AUTHORIZATION TO BE USED IN PLACE OF MY ORIGINAL SIGNATURE AND AUTHORIZE ANY HOLDER OF MEDICAL INFORMATION ABOUT ME TO RELEASE TO THE HEALTH CARE FINANCING ADMINISTRATION OR ITS AGENTS ANY INFORMATION NEEDED TO DETERMINE THESE BENEFITS OR THE BENEFITS PAYABLE FOR RELATED SERVICES.

Beryl Hawthorne
PATIENT/GUARDIAN SIGNATURE

9/24
DATE

Beryl Hawthorne

6/20 1 wk. post lap BP 120/70 LMP 6/9
TII sutures removed. Vertigo + weakness
CX - sutures

7/3 2 wks post lap BP 120/60 LMP 6/9
c/o abd. pain / pain in (L) hand
Ad: tender bilateral
Nordette 28's Return 1 mo

8/1 Pelvic Pain BP 110/80 LMP 7/9
Fatigue / Nausea / HA
Ad: no masses
Nordette x 1 mo CBC

9/15 mid pelvic pain BP 120/80
LMP 9/3
Ut: slight tender
ad: no masses
UGI, GB v12 BS

Andrew, Renee M.D.
St. Patrick Tower, Ste. 450
Payneville, TX 77777

The Pathology Laboratory
A Professional Medical Corporation

LABORATORY REPORT

PATIENT NAME	PATIENT ID	ROOM NO.	AGE	SEX	REFERRING PHYSICIAN
HAWTHORNE, BERYL			18	F	BENNATA

PAGE	REQUISITION NO.	ACCESSION NO.	LAB REF. #	COLLECTION DATE & TIME	LOG-IN-DATE	REPORT DATE	& TIME
1	5872579X	913122L		04/21	04/21	04/21	10:05

CYTOLOGY REPORT: PAP

CLINICAL HISTORY: TO BE COMPLETED BY REFERRING PHYSICIAN

SPECIMEN SOURCE: ☐ CERVIX ☐ VCE ☐ ENDOCERVIX ☐ VAGINA ☐ OTHER

LMP 4/12 PARA GRAV Age first pregnancy

PRIOR PAP CLASS (circle) None I II III IV IV V DATE

☐ Pregnant
☐ Postpartum
☐ Post Abortion
☐ Post Menop
☐ Hysterectomy
☐ Recent Cautery
☐ Susp. Lesion
☐ Prior CA _______
☐ Others ______________________________

☐ Spotting
☐ Discharge
☐ Ectropion
☐ IUD
☐ BC Pills
☐ Hormone Rx
☐ Condyloma
☐ Herpes

	Normal	Abnormal
Lugol's	☐	☐
Colpo	☐	☐
Cx Bx	☐	☐
Cx Cone	☐	☐
D & C	☐	☐

MATURATION INDEX

☐ Marked Estrogen effect (more than 60% superficial cells)
☐ Moderate Estrogen Effect (25 % to 60% superficial cells)
☑ Slight Estrogen Effect (up to 25% superficial cells)
☐ No evident Estrogen Effect (more than 25% intermediate cells & no superficial cells)
☐ Atrophic Smear (more than 75% parabasal cells)

Cells Present:

☐ White blood cells
☐ Mixed bacteria
☐ B. Vaginalis
☐ Endometrials

☐ Red blood cells
☐ Fungus
☐ Histiocytes
☐ Endocervicals

☐ Trichomonads
☐ G. Vaginalis (Clue Cell)
☐ Others ______________

DIAGNOSIS:

__✓__ CLASS I — NO EVIDENCE OF DYSPLASIA OR MALIGNANCY

_____ CLASS II — BENIN ATYPIAS

- ☐ Reactive or inflammatory atypia
- ☐ Atypical squamous metaplasia
- ☐ Reparative atypia
- ☐ Condyloma
- ☐ Herpes

_____ CLASS III — DYSPLASIAS

- ☐ Mild Dysplasia (CIN I)
- ☐ Moderate Dysplasia (CIN II)

_____ CLASS IV — SEVERE DYSPLASIA/CARCINOMA IN SITU (CIN III)

_____ CLASS V — CARCINOMAS

_____ CLASS O — SMEAR UNSUITABLE FOR EVALUATION

COMMENTS:

CLINICAL PATHOLOGIST	DATE REPORTED	ROOM	ACCESSION NO.
[signature]	4/21		

WEST
CAL-CAM
HOSPITAL

REPORT OF OPERATION

NAME: HAWTHORNE, BERYL DATE: 6-15
SURGEON: BENNATA ASSISTANT:
PREOPERATIVE DIAGNOSIS: PELVIC PAIN/ ENDOMETREOSIS

POSTOPERATIVE DIAGNOSIS: HEMOPERITONEM IN THE CUL-DE-SAC OF THE PELVIC CAVITY
R OVARIAN ENDOMETREOSIS

OPERATION PERFORMED: LAPAROSCOPY, ASPIRATION OF CUL-DE-SAC FLUID FOR CYTOLOGY
PELVIC CAVITY IRRIGATION AND ASPIRATION

After consents were signed and appropriated premedication given the patient was brought to the Operating Room where she was prepped and draped in the dorsal lithotomy position. Perineal, vaginal, abdominal skin preparation consisted of Betadine scrub sponges followed by Betadine solution swabs. A catheter was inserted. The patient was draped in routine fashion and general anesthesia was administered by the nurse anesthetist. 1 cm. subumbilical skin incision was made and a Verres needle was introduced with a negative aspiration test. 2 liter pneumoperitoneum with carbon dioxide was established and primary trocar was inserted. Inspection of the pelvic cavity revealed the presence of a 10 cc. hemoperitoneum in the cul-de-sac and samples were obtained and submitted to pathology for evaluation. Right ovarian endometriosis was noted with no endometriomas present, however stippling of the ovary with multiple small powder implants was noted.

The remainder of the contents of the pelvic cavity were inspected and noted to be within normal limits. The laparoscope was withdrawn under direct visualization and pneumoperitoneum was allowed to escape. The subumbilical and second puncture site incisions were closed with 3-0 Vicryl deep sutures followed with 3-0 Vicryl subcutaneous sutures. Lap, sponge and needle count were noted to be correct times 2.

The patient was transferred to the Recovery Room in good condition with stable vital signs.

ESTIMATED BLOOD LOSS: 20cc.

Darby Bennata, M.D.
dd: 6-15
dt: 6-16
skb

WEST CAL-CAM HOSPITAL

RADIOLOGY REPORT

NAME:	Hawthorne, Beryl	X-RAY#:	98891	RADIOLOGIST #:	19780
AGE: 18	SEX: F	ROOM NO:	OP	DATE:	09-19
EXAMINATION:	GI	ATTENDING DR:	Bennata	PATIENT #:	BH8501

UPPER GI SERIES:

No abnormalities of the esophagus are demonstrated. There is pylorospasm present during fluoroscopy. No active ulceration was demonstrated in the stomach or duodenum.

IMPRESSION: Pylorospasms.

BWJ/tmg

Bryan W. James, M.D.

Initial Pregnancy Profile

Date: mo/day/yr 9/24

HOLLISTER® maternal/newborn RECORD SYSTEM

PATIENT IDENTIFICATION

Patient's name: Beryl Hawthorne

History Since LMP (✓)

Check and detail all positive findings below. Use reference numbers.

Item	✓	Detail
1. Headaches	☑	Hx of HAs
2. Nausea/vomiting	☑	1st month
3. Abdominal pain	☑	x1 last Monday x1 hour off + on (call if reoccurs)
4. Urinary complaints	☐	
5. Vaginal discharge	☑	creamy
6. Vaginal bleeding	☐	
7. Edema (specify area)	☐	
8. Febrile episode	☑	T100 (due to injured finger)
9. Rubella exposure	☐	
10. Other viral exposure	☐	
11. Radiation exposure	☐	
12. ______	☐	
13. ______	☐	

14. Contraception prior to conception None ☑

Type ______

Last used mo/day/yr ______

15. Nutritional Assessment

☒ Adequate ☐ Inadequate

☐ Nutritional counseling

Remarks: ______

16. Medications Since LMP

☐ None ☐ Exposure to drugs

Describe: Cara Fat antacid

Initial Physical Examination

Height ☐ Weight ☐ Pregravid weight ☐ B.P. ☐ / Pulse ☐

OPTIONAL

Check and detail all abnormal findings below. Use reference numbers.

SYSTEM	Normal	Abn	Detail
17. Skin	☑	☐	
18. EENT	☑	☐	
19. Mouth	☑	☐	
20. Neck	☑	☐	supple
21. Chest	☑	☐	clear
22. Breast	☑	☐	w/o mass
23. Heart	☑	☐	RR w/o murmur
24. Lungs	☑	☐	clear
25. Abdomen	☑	☐	
26. Musculoskeletal	☑	☐	
27. Extremities	☑	☐	
28. Neurologic	☑	☐	
Pelvic Examination			
29. Ext. genitalia	☑	☐	
30. Vagina	☑	☐	
31. Cervix	☑	☐	
32. Uterus (describe)	☑	☐	9/30 13 weeks
33. Adnexa	☑	☐	
34. Rectum	☑	☐	
35. Other	☑	☐	

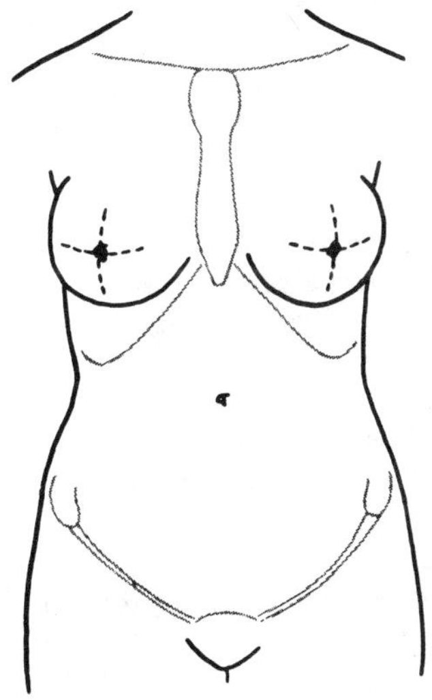

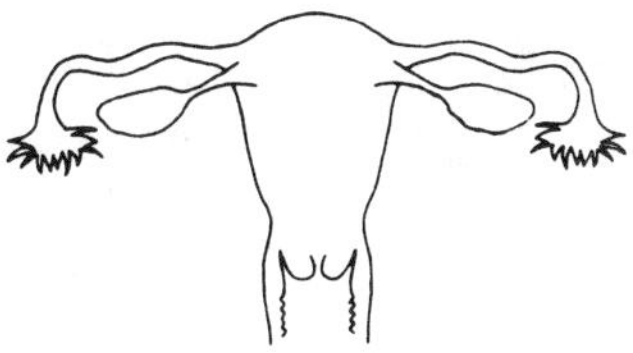

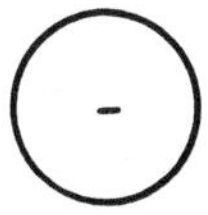

Bony Pelvis

36 Diag. conj. ______ 37 Shape sacrum ______ 38 S.S. notch ______ 39 Ischial spines ______

40 Pubic arch ______ 41 Trans. outlet ______ 42 Post sag. diam. ______ 43 Coccyx ______

44. Classification ☐ Gynecoid ☐ Android ☐ Anthropoid ☐ Platypelloid

45. Estimation ☐ Adequate ☐ Borderline ☐ Contracted

Exam done on mo/day/yr ______ by: ______

5871-4/86

Health History Summary

Date: mo/day/yr 9/24

HOLLISTER maternal/newborn RECORD SYSTEM

PATIENT IDENTIFICATION

Patient's name: Beryl Hawthorne
Home address: 1256 S. Vale Blvd. (STREET)
Payneville (CITY) TX (STATE) 77777 (ZIP)

Age: 20 Date of birth (mo/day/yr): 12/23 Race or ethnicity: Cau. Religion: Christian Marital status: S Years married: ____ Education: 12

Social Security number: ____ Occupation: ____ Work Tel. no. ____ Home Tel. no 555-7042

Alternate contact: Allie Hawthorne Relation to patient: gm. Work Tel. no. ____ Home Tel. no. 555-7484

Referring physician: ____ Attending physician: Dr. Darby Bennata

OPTIONAL FOR INSURANCE, ETC.

Medical History

Check and detail positive findings including date and place of treatment. Precede findings by reference number.

	Patient	Family	Findings
1. Congenital anomalies	☐	☑	sister (1 kidney)
2. Genetic diseases	☐	☐	
3. Multiple births	☐	☐	
4. Diabetes mellitus	☐	☐	
5. Malignancies	☐	☑	gm
6. Hypertension	☐	☐	
7. Heart disease	☐	☐	
8. Rheumatic fever	☐		
9. Pulmonary disease	☐	☑	gf (emphysema)
10. GI problems	☑		Ulcer (carafate Dx)
11. Renal disease	☑	☑	sister (chronic renal failure) Pt. donated kidney to sister.
12. Genitourinary tract problems	☐		
13. Abnormal uterine bleeding	☐		
14. Infertility	☐		
15. Venereal disease	☐	☐	denies hx herpes
16. Phlebitis, varicosities	☐		
17. Neurologic disorders	☐	☐	
18. Metabol./endocrine disorders	☐	☐	
19. Anemia/hemoglobinopathy	☑	☐	
20. Blood disorders	☐	☐	
21. Drug abuse	☐		
22. Smoking/alcohol use	☐		
23. Infectious diseases	☐		
24. Operations/accidents	☑		Kidney removed laparoscope
25. Allergies/meds sensitivity	☑		Dilantin
26. Blood transfusions	☐		
27. Other hospitalizations	☐		
28. ____	☐	☐	
29. ____	☐	☐	
30. **No known disease/problems**	☐	☐	

Preexisting Risk Guide

Indicates pregnancy/outcome at risk

31. ☐ Age <15 or >35
32. ☐ < 8th grade education
33. ☐ Cardiac disease (class I or II)
34. ☐ Tuberculosis, active
35. ☐ Chronic pulmonary disease
36. ☐ Thrombophlebitis
37. ☐ Endocrinopathy
38. ☐ Epilepsy (on medication)
39. ☐ Infertility (treated)
40. ☐ 2 abortions (spontaneous/induced)
41. ☐ ≥ 7 deliveries
42. ☐ Previous preterm or SGA infants
43. ☐ Infants ≥ 4,000 gms
44. ☐ Isoimmunization (ABO, etc.)
45. ☐ Hemorrhage during previous preg.
46. ☐ Previous preeclampsia
47. ☐ Surgically scarred uterus
48. ☐ Preg. without familial support
49. ☐ Second pregnancy in 12 months
50. ☐ Smoking (≥ 1 pack per day)
51. ☐ ____
52. ☐ ____
53. ☐ ____

Indicates pregnancy/outcome at high risk

54. ☐ Age ≥ 40
55. ☐ Diabetes mellitus
56. ☐ Hypertension
57. ☐ Cardiac disease (class III or IV)
58. ☒ Chronic renal disease (1 kidney)
59. ☐ Congenital/chromosomal anomalies
60. ☐ Hemoglobinopathies
61. ☐ Isoimmunization (Rh)
62. ☐ Alcohol or drug abuse
63. ☐ Habitual abortions
64. ☐ Incompetent cervix
65. ☐ Prior fetal or neonatal death
66. ☐ Prior neurologically damaged infant
67. ☐ Significant social problems
68. ☐ ____
69. ☐ ____
70. ☐ ____

Historical Risk Status

71. ☐ No risk factors noted
72. ☐ At risk
73. ☒ At **high** risk

Signature ____

Menstrual History

Onset	Cycle	Length	Amount	LMP mo/day/yr	quality
14 age	q. irreg. days	2-5 days	mod.	?/?	

Pregnancy History

Grav	Term	Pret	Abort	Live	EDC mo/day/yr
1					4/?

No.	Month/year	Sex	Weight at birth	Wks. gest.	Hrs. in labor	Type of delivery	Details of delivery: Include anesthesia and maternal or newborn complications. Use Risk Guide numbers where applicable.
1							
2							
3							
4							
5							
6							
7							
8							

Prenatal Flow Record

HOLLISTER® maternal/newborn RECORD SYSTEM

PATIENT IDENTIFICATION

Patient's name: Beryl Hawthorne

Historical Risk Factors and Assessment

Pt has 1 kidney

- [ ] 0 Has no known risk
- [ ] 1 Is "at risk"
- [x] 2 Is at **high risk**

Continuing Risk Assessment Guide (revise RISK STATUS)

Date	At risk factors	Date	**High risk** factors
/	Uterine/cervical malformation	/	Diabetes mellitus
/	Suspect pelvis	/	Hypertension
/	Rh negative (nonsensitized)	/	Thrombophlebitis
/	Anemia (Hct <30%:Hgb <10%)	/	Herpes (type 2)
/	Venereal disease	/	Rh sensitization
/	Acute pyelonephritis	/	Uterine bleeding
/	Failure to gain weight	/	Hydramnios
/	Abnormal presentation	/	Severe preeclampsia
/	Postterm pregnancy	/	Fetal growth retardation
/	Alcohol use	/	Premature rupt. membranes
/		/	Multiple pregnancy (preterm)
/		/	Alcohol and drug abuse
/		/	
/		/	

Initial Prenatal Screen / **Additional Lab Findings**

Initial Prenatal Screen	Date: mo/day/yr	Test	Date	Result	Date	Result
Hct/Hgb	36.5/12.4	Hct/Hgb	2/19	30.6/10.3	/	
Patient's Blood type and Rh	AB+	Blood sugar	/		/	
Antibody	Neg.	Antibody	/		/	
Serology	NR	Herpes	3/5	Neg	/	
Rubella titer	immune	Bacteriuria	/		/	
Urinalysis micro			/		/	
Pap test	9/8 no changes		/		/	
Cervical culture	GC neg	Strep	9/30	Neg	3/4	Neg
HBSAG	Neg	HIV	9/30	Neg	/	

LMP mo/day/yr 7/1 | EDC mo/day/yr 4/2 07 | Quickening date mo/day/yr

Medication Sensitivity ☐ None known or: Dilantin

- ☐ Initial prenatal instructions
- ☐ Attends prenatal classes
- ☐ Do herpes culture
- ☐ Do antenatal RhoGam
- ☐ For sterilization
- ☐ Circumcision
- ☐ Needs rubella vaccine
- ☐ Breast ☐ Bottle feeding

Amniocentesis
Explained on mo / day
☐ Accepted ☐ Rejected by patient

VBAC or C-Section
☐ OR records reviewed
Explained on mo / day
☐ Candidate for VBAC
☐ For Cesarean section

G T | T | Pt | A | L

Age 20

Weight Pre-gravid: /

Visit date 19__	Weight this visit	Blood pressure Base line	Urine protein	Urine Sugar	Est. weeks gestation (dates/size)	Fundal height	Fetal heart rate/quadrant	Edema			RISK STATUS (0, 1, 2)	Baby's physician	Return visit	Sig
/		/			/		+					denies Hx herpes		
9/28	DC c/o pain	Carafate off on sat-sun			/	desires to wait till	+			ok		ō thursday for US V.D. Dr. Bennata Farah LPN		
RF 9/30	147	110/70	tr	-	13/3	13 wks	+	-				pain L. abd. during night strep, ~~pap, GC~~ HIV drawn U/S		DB
10/5	fell down today - hit knees 1st no pains @ this time											notify office if pain, spotting, cramping occurs Farah LPN		
10/29	frequent pressure					BA						Bun CV ordered - Duricef 500 q 12 x 10 days		
11/3	states unable to buy Duricef will try Keftabs											Keftabs 500 ī q 8 hrs x 10 days Farah (U/A = mod bact.)		
11/6	146	110/80	tr	-	/	18 wks	⊕ 144	-				Rev u/a a lot of cramping	U/A 11/17	DB
RF 20 wks 11/17	147	123/70	-	-	/	20	+ 136	-				cramping ↓ abd. x 2 wks, frequent urination Keftabs 500 #20 tid x 10 d	10 d	DB
11/30	146	120/80	tr	-	/	20	+ 136	-				no appetite ↓ BA shooting pains Ⓡ side	1 wk	DB
/		/			/		+					BUNC		
12/3	cold, congested, Sudafed not helping request antibiotics											VCK 250mg q 6 x 8 days Farah LPN		
12/7	N/S		Pt		Ⓡ		12-10							
12/9	RF	Hydrocodone #30 ī q 4-6 hrs prn pain												Physician's signature: Farah LPN

Prenatal Flow Record (Continuation)

HOLLISTER maternal/newborn RECORD SYSTEM

PATIENT IDENTIFICATION

Patient's name: Beryl Hawthorne

G	T	Pt	A	L	Weight pregravid	LMP (mo/day/yr)	EDC (mo/day/yr)	Quickening date (mo/day/yr)
1					1	7/1	4/2 (U/S) 4/7	

Age: 20

Pt has 1 kidney

	Visit date 19__	Weight this visit	Blood pressure	Urine protein	Urine sugar	Est. weeks gestation (dates/size)	Fundal height	Fetal heart rate/quadrant	Edema	Risk status (0 1 2)	Notes	Return visit	Sig.
23	12/10	144	94/70	tr	-	23/23	22	⊕ 156	—		Fe, vit D to ER; mild ↓BA	2 wk	[illegible]
26	12/30	152	120/68	tr	-	/	25	⊕ 156	—		poss. yeast infection; ↓BA on Ⓡ side		
	1/4	refill Hydrocodone #30 ‒ q 4-6 hrs prn pain — Faun LPN											
28	1/14	153	126/78	tr	-	27/27	27	⊕ 152	—		not urinating as often; Sunday 5 contractions in 30 min	3 wk	DB
	1/21	Hydrocodone #10 ‒ q 4-6 hrs prn pain K+B Sulphur v.o. Dr. Darby / Faun LPN											
	/	Pt asked if ok to go to Amarillo TX 24-28 hr drive. Advised risk and explained Dr. ODF T. Faun LPN											
	1/27	weak, no energy, N+V. Bottom of stomach sore, hip hurts, Ⓡ side feels bones are coming apart. Pain in shoulder pain heartburn. TO office T. Faun LPN											
31 1/2	1/27	151	122/78	tr	-	/	27	⊕ 168	sm		weak, N+V, hips hurt Ⓡ side pain; FHT's 168 abd real sore sharp pain vag. area		
	2/2							+			U/S P-12 (Bum C/)	Mon.	DB
	2/2	(148)	112/82	tr	-	/	(28)	⊕ 116	sm	nausea vomiting	FHTs 116 ↑abd sore from coughing - felt weak; coughing since Fri; Ⓡ side pain		
	/							+			Robitussin AC		DB
	2/9	? leakage of fluids, freq. urination, weak, shaky, vomiting, cold sweats, vomiting, mouth watering; refill Hydrocodone									TO OB		
	/							+					
33	2/12	150	128/90	tr	-	/	(28)	⊕ 152	sm		tender abd; cough Ⓡ side pain	4 wk	DB
	/					/		+			u/s y siz c data		
34	2/19	154	130/78	tr	-	33/30	(28)	⊕ 120	—		a lot of pressure FAD u/s H+H	10 d	DB
	/					/		+			↑ wn do u/s		
	3/1	Refill Hydrocodone #30 ‒ p.o. q 4-6 hrs prn pain — Faun LPN											
	3/4	153	114/80	tr	-	36/	31	⊕ 140			has felt no movement today; pressure rib cage area sore strep herpes		
	/							+			BUN, Cr, [illegible] NST	1 wk	DB
	3/5	Ⓛ eye swollen, yellow drainage, NST this AM - Cortis. Opth 3 gtts in affected eye gtts - Faun											
	3/11	154	122/80	tr	-	37/37	33	⊕	sm		Pb contracting NST	1 wk	DB
	3/15							+			Repeat NST Tues / or Wed		
	/			/		/		+					
	/			/		/		+					

Physician's Signature

PRENATAL FLOW RECORD (Cont.)

5873-4/86

MATERNAL RECORD COPY

WEST
CAL-CAM
HOSPITAL

HISTORY SHEET

NAME: Hawthorne, Beryl DATE: 11-21 ROOM NO.:
ATTENDING PHYSICIAN: Bennata
CHIEF COMPLAINT: Severe right flank pain
Right lower quandrant pain

PRESENT ILLNESS:

The patient is a 20 year old G-I P-O whose last menstrual period was 7-1 EDC 4-11. The patient has a history of being a left nephrectomy donor for her sister. The patient has a history of pain in her right flank region which extends down into her right lower quadrant. She is admitted for pain relief and evaluation of pain.

PAST HISTORY:

SURGICAL: See present illness.
MEDICAL: The patient has a history of gastric ulcer in September.
ALLERGIES: Dilantin.
CHILDHOOD: Usual illnesses.
FAMILY HISTORY: Positive for cancer, emphysema, renal disease.
SOCIAL HISTORY: The patient denies use of ethanol or tobacco.

ROS:

GENERAL: No chills, fever, night sweats.
HEENT: No tinnitus, diplopia, epistaxis.
CARDIORESPIRATORY: Denies chest pain, PND or DOE.
GI: No nausea, vomiting, diarrhea or melena.
GU: See present illness.
NM: Noncontributory.

Darby Bennata, M.D.
dd: 11-21
dt: 11-21
tmf

WEST
CAL-CAM
HOSPITAL

PHYSICAL EXAMINATION

NAME: Hawthorne, Beryl DATE: 11-21 ROOM NO.:
ATTENDING PHYSICIAN: Bennata

VITAL SIGNS: TEMP: 97 PULSE: 75 RESP: 20 BP: 109/63
GENERAL: The patient is alert and oriented to time and place, and in no apparent distress.

SKIN: Good turgor, texture and coloration.

HEENT: Normocephalic, PERRLA, EOM's intact, fundi benign, tympanic membranes, external ear canals clear bilaterally.

NECK: Supple, full range of motion. No lymphadenopathy or thyromegaly. Pharynx within normal limits, no bruits or JVD noted.

CHEST: Clear to auscultation and percussion, no rales, rubs, or rhonchi. Good symmetry with good inspiratory effort, no gross deformity.

HEART: Regular rhythm without murmur or gallop. S1 and S2 within normal limits. PMI at the left intercostal space and in the midclavicular line.

ABDOMEN: Tender to deep palpation in the right lower quadrant. Positive costovertebral angle tenderness is noted on the right.

PELVIC EXAMINATION: Reveals a cervix is long closed and posterior.

EXTREMITIES: No cyanosis, clubbing or edema. Full range of motion in all joints. Distal pulses are equal.

NEUROLOGICAL: Cranial nerves 2 through 12 are grossly intact. Deep tendon reflexes are 2+ out 3+ and bilaterally equal. No abnormal reflexes are elicited.

IMPRESSION: INTRAUTERINE PREGNANCY UNDELIVERED
SEVERE RIGHT LOWER QUADRANT AND RIGHT FLANK PAIN
PROBABLE OVARIAN VEIN SYNDROME

D Bennata

Darby Bennata, M.D.
dd: 11-21
dt: 11-22
tmf

WEST
CAL-CAM
HOSPITAL

PROGRESS NOTES

NAME: HAWTHORNE, BERYL DATE: 11-22

The patient complains of right costovertebral angle tenderness and pain with no difficulty urinating. She denies any chills or hematuria. Exam reveals minimal costovertebral angle tenderness to deep palpation in the right costovertebral angle area.

IMPRESSION: Rule out ovarian vein syndrome.

PLANS: Continue IV antibiotics and ambulate. Urology consult.

Darby Bennata, M.D.
dd: 11-22
dt: 11-23
tmf

WEST CAL-CAM HOSPITAL

PROGRESS NOTES

NAME: HAWTHORNE, BERYL DATE: 11-26

The patient's residual urine was 100 cc., however, she voided another 125 cc. following catheterization. She did relate some bleeding after catheterization. She continues to experience urinary frequency. She has not attempted the knee chest position for her pain and the pain during the night was unrelieved by rolling from side to side. Repeat urinalysis reveals 1 to 2 white cells, occasional bacteria, with a specific gravity of 1.015.

I discussed the etiology of the CVA discomfort with the patient, stating that I did not believe that she had obstructive disease with a 24 hour urine output yesterday greater than 3 liters. Regarding her lower urinary symptoms of frequency and constant urge to void, I advised her this is likely related to the enlargement of her uterus and on listening to her describe again her urine flow, which is relatively forceful and easy, I do not feel she is retaining significant residual urine. Because of the bleeding and difficulty with catheterization, I choose not to repeat her residual urine. We further discussed the use of anticholinergics and antispasmotics, which may improve this pattern of voiding after her pregnancy. She states that this pattern of voiding existed prior to her pregnancy.

Regarding fluid intake, which was a conversational discussion between the two of us, I advised her that forcing fluids is not necessary under normal circumstances, meaning when she is not running a high fever and dehydrating or sweating profusely -- such as in yard work during the summer. I advised her to drink, certainly, what she is thirsty for, but not to impose a minimum goal of 10 to 12 glasses of water a day when there were no unusual circumstances and she did not perceive thirst. We discussed briefly diabetes insipidus, though I did not feel this was a likely diagnosis and would be reluctant to treat her with Pitressin during pregnancy. Tests for diabetes insipidus are feasible post delivery.

I would additionally avoid alpha adrenergic medication, such as Sudafed.

Darby Bennata, M.D.
dd: 11-22
dt: 11-23
tmf

WEST
CAL-CAM
HOSPITAL

DISCHARGE SUMMARY

NAME: Hawthorne, Beryl ADMIT DATE: 11-21 DISCHARGE DATE: 11-26

BRIEF HISTORY: The patient is a 20 year old G-1 P-0 with a history of costovertebral angle tenderness on the right which is intermittent. She is admitted for evaluation for possible urolithiasis and/or renal obstruction. The patient has a history of having a unilateral right kidney, being a donor for her sister with the left.

PERTINENT PHYSICAL FINDINGS: Alert oriented female in no acute distress except for right costovertebral angle pain.

PERTINENT LABORATORY AND X-RAY FINDINGS: Urinalysis reveals 20 to 25 red blood cells per high power field and 2 to 4 whites per high power field. Urine cultures were sterile.

HOSPITAL COURSE: The patient was admitted and put on analgesics and IV antibiotics. She was seen in consultation by Dr. Perkins who recommended some changes in her voiding pattern fluid intact. Following this, her pain was noted to gradually subside, and she was discharged on 11-26. Medications on discharge include iron and vitamins as prescribed previously, Tylenol #3 po q 4 hours prn pain.

FINAL DIAGNOSIS: INTRAUTERINE PREGNANCY UNDELIVERED
PROBABLE OVARIAN VEIN SYNDROME
ABNORMAL VOIDING PATTERN

Darby Bennata, M.D.
dd: 11-26
dt: 11-27
tmf

WEST CAL-CAM HOSPITAL

PROGRESS NOTES

NAME: HAWTHORNE, BERYL DATE: 12-20

HOSPITAL DAY #2

Vital signs are stable. Abdomen is soft. No CVA or rebound. The patient complains of tenderness in the right lower quadrant. Pelvic examination reveals a cervix which is long closed and posterior.

PLANS: Continue pain medications and bedrest.

HOSPITAL DAY #4

Vital signs are stable. Urine output is adequate. Chest is clear to auscultation and percussion. Fetal movement is palpable. No CVA or rebound is noted. No tenderness to deep palpitation in the right lower quadrant.

Darby Bennata, M.D.
dd: 12-22
dt: 12-23
tmf

WEST
CAL-CAM
HOSPITAL

DISCHARGE SUMMARY

NAME: Hawthorne, Beryl ADMIT DATE: 12-19 DISCHARGE DATE: 12-24

BRIEF HISTORY: The patient is a 20 year old G-1 P-0 whose last menstrual period was 7-1 EDC 4-11. The patient has a history of ovarian vein syndrome and right lower quadrant pain and right flank pain with abnormal voiding pattern. The patient presents with a chief complaint of return of urinary symptoms including dysuria, post-voiding spasm and right lower quadrant pain. She was admitted for evaluation and pain relief.

PERTINENT PHYSICAL FINDINGS: Tenderness to deep palpitation of right lower quadrant and positive costovertebral angle tenderness on the right.

PERTINENT LABORATORY AND X-RAY FINDINGS: Fetal ultrasound reveals an EDC of 4-4. Renal ultrasound reveals no abnormality of the right kidney.

HOSPITAL COURSE: The patient was admitted and placed on pain medication and oral antibiotics to which she showed a gradual response with a clearing of her symptoms. She was discharged on 12-24 to be followed in the office on 12-30. Discharge medications include Mepergan Fortes 1 po q 4 hours prn pain.

FINAL DIAGNOSIS: INTRAUTERINE PREGNANCY UNDELIVERED
PYELONEPHRITIS
CYSTITIS
RIGHT OVARIAN VEIN SYNDROME

Darby Bennata, M.D.
dd: 12-24
dt: 12-25
tmf

SHORT STAY ADMISSION

WEST
CAL-CAM
HOSPITAL

NAME: HAWTHORNE, BERYL ADMIT DATE: 02-09 DISCHARGE DATE: 2-10

HISTORY OF PRESENT ILLNESS:
The patient is a 21 year old G-1 P-0 with a history of recurrent pelvic pain during this pregnancy. The patient presents with a chief complaint of vaginal leakage of clear fluid on a frequent basis on the day of admission. The patient states that the fluid leakage was to the point where it required use of a sanitary pad. The patient also complained of intermittent uterine contractions with uterine irritability.

ROS:

GENERAL:	No chills, fever, night sweats.
HEENT:	No tinnitus, diplopia, epistaxis.
CARDIORESPIRATORY:	Denies chest pain, PND or DOE.
GI:	No nausea, vomiting, diarrhea, or melena.
GU:	See present illness.
NM:	Noncontributory.

PHYSICAL EXAMINATION:

VITAL SIGNS:	BP; PULSE; RESP; TEMP;
GENERAL:	The patient is an alert, oriented female in no acute distress.
HEENT:	Normocephalic, PERRLA, EOM's intact, fundi benign.
CHEST:	Clear to auscultation and percussion, no rales, rubs or rhonchi. Good symmetry, good inspiratory effort.
HEART:	Regular rhythm without murmur, gallop, click or rub. S1 and S2 within normal limits. PMI left fifth intercostal space in midclavicular line.
BREASTS:	The patient has engorged and extremely tender breasts with no evidence of abscess. She shows no skin changes over her breasts other than erythema.
ABDOMEN:	Soft.
PELVIC EXAM:	Reveals a cervix which is a dimple and the vertex is at a +1 station.
EXTREMITIES:	No cyanosis, clubbing or edema. Full range of motion in all joints.
NEUROLOGICAL:	Cranial nerves 2-12 grossly intact. Deep tendon reflexes 2+ out of 3+ and bilaterally equal. No abnormal reflexes are elicited.

PROGRESS: The patient was admitted for observation for possible preterm labor and rupture of membranes. She was noted to not have any further leakage or contractions. Following this, she was discharged on Brethine 2.5 PO q 6 hours and iron and vitamins as prescribed previously.

OPERATION: NONE

CONDITION: The patient is eating and ambulating with no complaints of pain, chills or fever.

DIAGNOSIS: INTRAUTERINE PREGNANCY UNDELIVERED
POSSIBLE PREMATURE RUPTURE OF MEMBRANES

Darby Bennata, M.D.
dd: 2-10
dt: 2-11
tmf

WEST
CAL-CAM
HOSPITAL

RADIOLOGY REPORT

NAME: Hawthorne, Beryl X-RAY#: 98921 RADIOLOGIST #: 19780
AGE: 21 SEX: F ROOM NO: 4110 DATE: 03-17
EXAMINATION: CT T/S & L/S ATTENDING DR: Bennata PATIENT #: BH8501

CT SCAN OF THE LOWER THORACIC AND LUMBAR SPINE:

Air is seen in a portion of the epidural space which is probably due to the epidural anesthesia which was administered one day earlier. A significant epidural hematoma is not identified. IF SYMPTOMS PERSIST, A SMALL AMOUNT OF OMNIPAQUE 180 CAN BE INTRODUCED INTO THE SUBARACHNOID SPACE AND THE CT REPEATED WHICH WOULD BETTER OUTLINE THE SUBARACHNOID SPACE AND PROVIDE BETTER CONTRAST MATERIAL TO SEPARATE THE EPIDURAL SPACE FROM THE SUBARACHNOID SPACE.

IMPRESSION:

CT scan of the lower thoracic and lumbar spine reveal some minimal amount of air in the epidural space from the recent epidural anesthesia. A significant epidural hematoma is not visualized. Better contrast could be obtained with some contrast material introduced into the subarachnoid space. This may be indicated clinically.

BWJ/tmf
dt: 3-17

Bryan W. James, M.D.

H

B

L
E
Lindale, Evelyn Acct.# EL4232 Dr. Thomas

Patient Information

PLEASE PRINT

PATIENT NAME Evelyn Lindale AGE 49

ADDRESS Box 610, RR6 BIRTHDATE Feb 21

Painesville, TX 11111 SEX F

SOCIAL SECURITY 666-33-2222 MARITAL STATUS M. PHONE (713) 973-1397

EMPLOYER Homemaker PHONE ( )

Please complete if patient is a minor or another party will be responsible for bill.

RESPONSIBLE PARTY self RELATION

ADDRESS (IF DIFFERENT)

SOCIAL SECURITY BIRTHDATE PHONE ( )

TYPE OF COVERAGE: MEDICARE MEDICAID GROUP SELF PAY (OTHER)

MEDICARE PART A PART B

NAME ON CARD MEDICARE NUMBER

MEDICAID

NAME ON CARD MEDICAID NUMBER EFFECTIVE DATE

PRIMARY HEALTH INSURANCE Bell Insurance Co.

COMPANY NAME ADDRESS

Bill Lindale 76-32437

POLICY HOLDER POLICY NUMBER GROUP NUMBER

SECONDARY HEALTH INSURANCE

COMPANY NAME ADDRESS

POLICY HOLDER POLICY NUMBER GROUP NUMBER

I REQUEST THAT PAYMENT OF AUTHORIZED INSURANCE BENEFITS BE MADE EITHER TO ME OR ON MY BEHALF TO THE UNDERSIGNED PROVIDER FOR SERVICES FURNISHED ME BY THAT PHYSICIAN. I PERMIT A COPY OF THIS AUTHORIZATION TO BE USED IN PLACE OF MY ORIGINAL SIGNATURE AND AUTHORIZE ANY HOLDER OF MEDICAL INFORMATION ABOUT ME TO RELEASE TO THE HEALTH CARE FINANCING ADMINISTRATION OR ITS AGENTS ANY INFORMATION NEEDED TO DETERMINE THESE BENEFITS OR THE BENEFITS PAYABLE FOR RELATED SERVICES.

Evelyn Lindale Jan. 31

PATIENT/GUARDIAN SIGNATURE DATE

E. Ewidale
1-31

49 Y/O WF for evaluation of a mole on her Ⓛ cheek which has recently become pruritic. lesion has not changed in appearance + otherwise is asymptomatic.

PE: see diagram

Imp: nevus

Rec: observation; RTC prn any significant change in lesion.

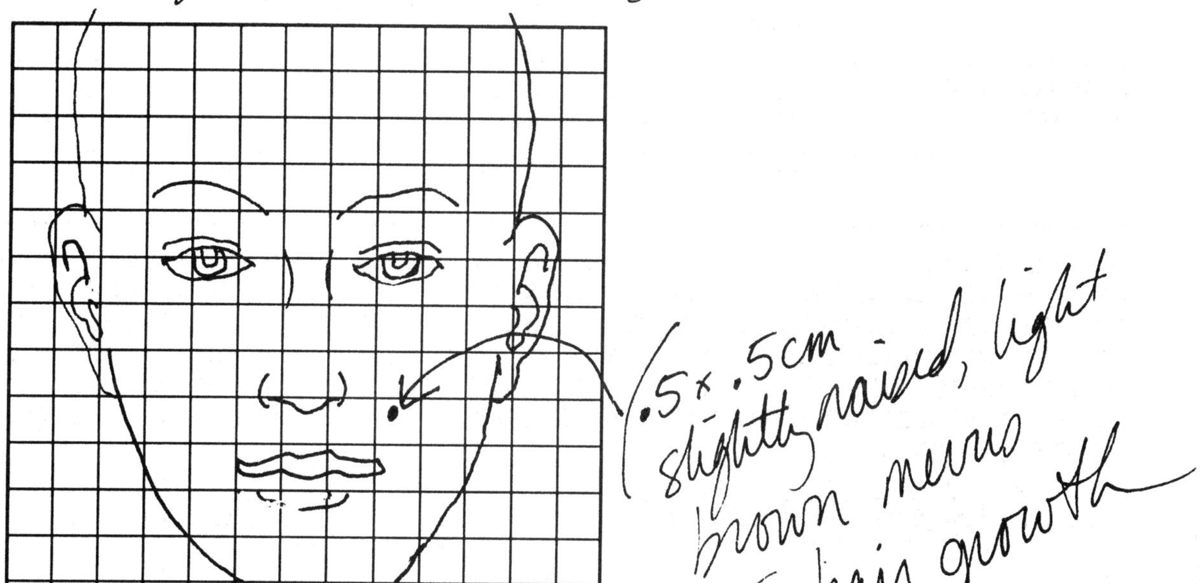

L

E

S
B
Saman, Bernice Acct. # BS8505 Dr. Bennata

Patient Information

PLEASE PRINT

PATIENT NAME Bernice Saman   AGE 20

ADDRESS 519 Shady Lane #212   BIRTHDATE 9/4

Payneville, Texas   SEX F

SOCIAL SECURITY 333-22-4444   MARITAL STATUS M   PHONE (713) 973-7357

EMPLOYER MEDBOOKS   PHONE (800) 413-7357

Please complete if patient is a minor or another party will be responsible for bill.

RESPONSIBLE PARTY ____________________ RELATION ________

ADDRESS (IF DIFFERENT) ____________________

SOCIAL SECURITY __________ BIRTHDATE __________ PHONE (   ) __________

TYPE OF COVERAGE: MEDICARE MEDICAID (GROUP) SELF PAY OTHER

MEDICARE ____________________ PART A PART B

NAME ON CARD MEDICARE NUMBER

MEDICAID ____________________

NAME ON CARD MEDICAID NUMBER EFFECTIVE DATE

PRIMARY HEALTH INSURANCE BlueCross/BlueShield of Texas

COMPANY NAME ADDRESS

Joe Saman 999J5888

POLICY HOLDER POLICY NUMBER GROUP NUMBER

SECONDARY HEALTH INSURANCE ____________________

COMPANY NAME ADDRESS

POLICY HOLDER POLICY NUMBER GROUP NUMBER

I REQUEST THAT PAYMENT OF AUTHORIZED INSURANCE BENEFITS BE MADE EITHER TO ME OR ON MY BEHALF TO THE UNDERSIGNED PROVIDER FOR SERVICES FURNISHED ME BY THAT PHYSICIAN. I PERMIT A COPY OF THIS AUTHORIZATION TO BE USED IN PLACE OF MY ORIGINAL SIGNATURE AND AUTHORIZE ANY HOLDER OF MEDICAL INFORMATION ABOUT ME TO RELEASE TO THE HEALTH CARE FINANCING ADMINISTRATION OR ITS AGENTS ANY INFORMATION NEEDED TO DETERMINE THESE BENEFITS OR THE BENEFITS PAYABLE FOR RELATED SERVICES.

Bernice Saman   5-2

PATIENT/GUARDIAN SIGNATURE   DATE

RADIOLOGY REPORT

WEST
CAL-CAM
HOSPITAL

NAME: Saman, Bernice	X-RAY#: 58395	RADIOLOGIST #: 8015
AGE: 20 SEX: F	ROOM NO: OP	DATE: 5-7
EXAMINATION: OB U/S	ATTENDING DR: Bennata	PATIENT #: BS8505

OB ULTRASOUND:
A gestational sac is identified intrauterine. A heartbeat is identified within the gestational sac. From the size of the gestational sac which averages 20.4 mm, the gestational age is estimated to be 6.5 weeks. Using that data, the EDC is projected to be 28 December. Right ovary is normal size. Left ovary is not as well seen, but no mass or cyst is identified.

IMPRESSION: Intrauterine gestational sac with a heartbeat. From sac size, EDC is projected to be 28 December.

STD/tmg
dt: 5-7

Scott Davis, M.D.

Stevens, Sam M.D.
St. Patrick Tower, Ste. 450
Payneville, TX 77777

The Pathology Laboratory
A Professional Medical Corporation

LABORATORY REPORT

PATIENT NAME	PATIENT ID	ROOM NO.	AGE	SEX	REFERRING PHYSICIAN
SAMAN, BERNICE			20	F	BENNATA

PAGE	REQUISITION NO.	ACCESSION NO.	LAB REF.#	COLLECTION DATE & TIME	LOG-IN-DATE	REPORT DATE	& TIME
1	3983579X	875225L		07/12	07/12	07/16	14:39

REPORT STATUS FINAL TEST	RESULT IN RANGE	RESULT OUT OF RANGE	UNITS	REFERENCE RANGE	SITE CODE
ALPHA-FETOPROTEIN, MATERNAL SERUM SEE BAYLOR REPORT	NG/ML				
MSAFP	41.30		NG/ML		
GESTATIONAL AGE	16.0				
MULTIPLE OF MEDIAN					
PATIENT WEIGHT	196		LBS		
PATIENT RACE	CAUCASIAN				
DIABETES	NO				
ADJ MULTIPLE MEDIAN	1.57				
MSAFP RISK OPEN NTD	1 IN 4513				
AGE RISK DOWN SYND	1 IN 2240				

INTERPRETATION:

SERUM MSAFP IS WITHIN NORMAL RANGE FOR STATED GESTATIONAL AGE AND MATERNAL WEIGHT.

These results are baased on patient data above. The interpretation is dependent on the accuracy of this information. All information should be current as of specimin date. Any corrections or additions should be reported to our office for recalculation. A normal result does not guarantee a normal fetus. Low serum AFP will detect only 20-30% of Down Syndrome Pregnancies.

>>END OF REPORT<<

RADIOLOGY REPORT

WEST
CAL-CAM
HOSPITAL

NAME: Saman, Bernice
AGE: 20 SEX: F
EXAMINATION: OB U/S

X-RAY#: 58101
ROOM NO: OP
ATTENDING DR: Bennata

RADIOLOGIST #: 8015
DATE: 8-27
PATIENT #: BS8505

OB ULTRASOUND:
The parietal diameter, head circumference, abdominal circumference, and femoral length measurements at 54.7, 199.8, 172.2, and 38.8 respectively, corresponding to gestational ages of 22.7, 22.1, 22.2, and 22.5 weeks. Using a computed mean average of 22.1 + or - 1.4 weeks the EDC is predicted to 31 December. The estimated fetal weight is 515 grams + or - 69 grams. This is in the 45 percentile range for ultrasound parameters. A single fetus is present in a breech presentation with normal cardiac motion and a four chamber heart. The placenta is located anteriorly and is judged to be a Grade I placenta. The umbilical cord contains three vessels. The amniotic fluid is within normal limits. The fetal bladder is visualized. The fetal kidneys are not well seen. The fetal stomach and fetal spine are judged to be within normal limits.

IMPRESSION: EDC is predicted to be 31 December.

STD/tmg
dd: 8-27
dt: 8-27
dsrp: 8-27

Scott Davis, M.D.

WEST CAL-CAM HOSPITAL

RADIOLOGY REPORT

NAME:	Saman, Bernice	X-RAY#:	58254	RADIOLOGIST #:	8015
AGE: 21	SEX: F	ROOM NO:	7002	DATE:	11-13
EXAMINATION:	OB U/S	ATTENDING DR:	Bennata	PATIENT #:	BS8505

OB ULTRASOUND:

A single fetus was identifeid in vertex presentation. There was fetal motion and heart beat. The placenta is located anteriorly without evidence of abruptio. The placenta is Grade III. The amount of amniotic fluid appears to be within normal limits. Gestational age was estimated from measurements of BPD, HC, AC and FL. These were 83, 300, 293 and 65 mms. respectively suggesting gestational ages of 33.3, 33.2, 33.3 and 33.6 weeks respectively. Overall gestational age is estimated at 33.0 plus or minus 2.4 weeks with EDC of January 1.

STD/tmg
dd: 11-13
dt: 11-13
dsrp: 11-13

Scott Davis, M.D.

WEST CAL-CAM HOSPITAL

DISCHARGE SUMMARY

NAME: SAMAN, BERNICE ADMIT DATE: 11-13 DISCHARGE DATE: 11-14

HISTORY OF PRESENT ILLNESS: The patient is a 21 year old S-1 P-0 whose EDC is 12-28. The patient presents with a chief complaint of intermittent uterine contractions at home and states that she has felt tightening in her lower abdomen and upper fundus on the day of admission. The patient denies any leakage of fluid per vagina but described intermittent staining on her underwear with a pink discharge. The patent states that she has felt good fetal movement and denies any dysuria or hematuria.

PERTINENT LABORATORY AND X-RAY FINDINGS: OB ultrasound reveals the presence of a single fetus in vertex presentation with an EDC of Jan. 1 at 33 weeks gestation.

HOSPITAL COURSE: The patient was admitted and placed on the fetal monitor with follow-up for vaginal bleeding including a hematocrit and ultrasound. The patient was begun on Brethine tablets orally 2.5 PO q 6 hours and was instructed to the office on Wednesday following discharge for post-hospital follow-up.

FINAL DIAGNOSIS: INTRAUTERINE PREGNANCY UNDELIVERED, 33 WEEKS
PRETERM LABOR

Darby Bennata, M.D.
dd: 11-14
dt: 11-15
mc

WEST CAL-CAM HOSPITAL

SHORT STAY ADMISSION

NAME: SAMAN, BERNICE ADMIT DATE: 11-28 DISCHARGE DATE: 11-29

HISTORY OF PRESENT ILLNESS:
The patient is a 21 year old female G-1 P-0 whose EDC is 12-28 who presents with a chief complaint of intermittent contractions. The patient has been maintained on Amoxicillin 250 PO tid for urinary tract infection. The patient presents with a chief complaint of intermittent contractions and low back pain.

ROS:

GENERAL:	No chills, fever, night sweats.
HEENT:	No tinnitus, diplopia, epistaxis.
CARDIORESPIRATORY:	Denies chest pain, PND or DOE/
GI:	No nausea, vomiting, diarrhea or melena.
GU:	See present illness.
NM:	Noncontributory.

PHYSICAL EXAMINATION:

VITAL SIGNS:	BP; PULSE; RESP; TEMP;
GENERAL:	The patient is an alert oriented female in no acute distress.
HEENT:	Normocephalic, PERRLA, EOM's intact, fundi benign.
CHEST:	Clear to auscultation and percussion, no rales, rubs, or rhonchi. Good symmetry, good inspiratory effort.
HEART:	Regular rhythm without murmur, gallop, click or rub. S1 and S2 within normal limits. PMI left fifth intercostal space in midclavicular line.
ABDOMEN:	Soft. Gravid uterus approximately 36 weeks size.
PELVIC EXAM:	Cervix is a dimple and still firm.
EXTREMITIES:	No cyanosis, clubbing, or edema. Full range of motion is all joints.
NEUROLOGICAL:	Cranial nerves 2-12 grossly intact. Deep tendon reflexes 2+ out of 3+ and bilaterally equal. No abnormal reflexes are elicited.

PROGRESS: The patient was admitted and observed overnight. Contractions were noted to gradually subside and she was discharged.

OPERATION: NONE
CONDITION: The patient is eating and ambulating.

DIAGNOSIS: INTRAUTERINE PREGNANCY UNDELIVERED
BRAXTON -HICKS CONTRACTIONS

Darby Bennata, M.D.
dd: 11-29
dt: 11-30
mc

WEST
CAL-CAM
HOSPITAL

LABOR AND DELIVERY NOTE

NAME: Saman, Bernice

12-14

The patient is a 21 year old G-1 P-0 whose EDC is 12-28 who presents with a chief complaint of questionable rupture of membranes and was referred over by my office for evaluation. Nitrozine testing x 2 even after ambulation reveals no color change. The patient's cervix is soft 1 cm retrocessed. Diastolic blood pressure in the office was noted to be above 100; however, multiple repeat values in Labor and Delivery reveal it to be less than 90, in the 61 to 70 range. The patient is being discharged with precautions to return for rupture of membranes, headaches, and increased swelling. She is requested to follow-up in the office on Friday for blood pressure check and cervix evaluation.

Darby Bennata, M.D.
dd: 12-14
dt: 12-14
mc

S

B

S
T
Spitz, Terry Acct.# TS9012 Dr. T. Rassler

Patient Information

PLEASE PRINT

PATIENT NAME Jerry Spitz AGE 36

ADDRESS 2040 Homestead BIRTHDATE 8-58

Paynesville, TX 77777 SEX F

SOCIAL SECURITY 777-11-3333 MARITAL STATUS M PHONE (713) 773-7397

EMPLOYER self-employed PHONE ( )

Please complete if patient is a minor or another party will be responsible for bill.

RESPONSIBLE PARTY self RELATION

ADDRESS (IF DIFFERENT)

SOCIAL SECURITY BIRTHDATE PHONE ( )

TYPE OF COVERAGE: MEDICARE MEDICAID GROUP SELF PAY (OTHER)

MEDICARE PART A PART B

NAME ON CARD MEDICARE NUMBER

MEDICAID

NAME ON CARD MEDICAID NUMBER EFFECTIVE DATE

PRIMARY HEALTH INSURANCE BC/BS of Texas

COMPANY NAME ADDRESS

Jerry Spitz 777-11-3333

POLICY HOLDER POLICY NUMBER GROUP NUMBER

SECONDARY HEALTH INSURANCE Prudential

COMPANY NAME ADDRESS

John Spitz 342TP

POLICY HOLDER POLICY NUMBER GROUP NUMBER

I REQUEST THAT PAYMENT OF AUTHORIZED INSURANCE BENEFITS BE MADE EITHER TO ME OR ON MY BEHALF TO THE UNDERSIGNED PROVIDER FOR SERVICES FURNISHED ME BY THAT PHYSICIAN. I PERMIT A COPY OF THIS AUTHORIZATION TO BE USED IN PLACE OF MY ORIGINAL SIGNATURE AND AUTHORIZE ANY HOLDER OF MEDICAL INFORMATION ABOUT ME TO RELEASE TO THE HEALTH CARE FINANCING ADMINISTRATION OR ITS AGENTS ANY INFORMATION NEEDED TO DETERMINE THESE BENEFITS OR THE BENEFITS PAYABLE FOR RELATED SERVICES.

Jerry Spitz 3-11

PATIENT/GUARDIAN SIGNATURE DATE

Rassler, Tom M.D.
St. Patrick Tower, Ste. 450
Payneville, TX 77777

The Pathology Laboratory
A Professional Medical Corporation

LABORATORY REPORT

PATIENT NAME	PATIENT ID	ROOM NO.	AGE	SEX	REFERRING PHYSICIAN
SPITZ, TERRY			36	F	BENNATA

PAGE	REQUISITION NO.	ACCESSION NO.	LAB REF.#	COLLECTION DATE & TIME	LOG-IN-DATE	REPORT DATE	& TIME
1	3982170	875328L		03/11	03/11	03/15	4:41PM

REPORT STATUS: FINAL

TEST	RESULT IN RANGE	RESULT OUT OF RANGE	UNITS	REFERENCE RANGE	SITE CODE
ALPHA-FETOPROTEIN, MATERNAL SERUM					
MSAFP	38.5		NG/ML		
GESTATIONAL AGE	16				
MULTIPLE OF MEDIAN	1.1				
PATIENT WEIGHT	131		LBS		
PATIENT RACE	CAUCASIAN				
DIABETES	NO				
ADJ MULTIPLE MEDIAN	1.0				
MSAFP RISK OPEN NTD	1 IN 8829				
AGE RISK DOWN SYND	1 IN 213 - INCREASED RISK (SEE BELOW)				
MSAFP RISK DOWN SYND	SEE BELOW				

INTERPRETATION:

ALTHOUGH MSAFP IS WITHIN NORMAL LIMITS FOR STATED GESTATIONAL AGE AND DEMOGRAPHIC DATA PROVIDED, MATERNAL AGE IS 35 OR OLDER (SEE RECOMMENDATION BELOW).

THIS PATIENT IS 35 YEARS OF AGE OR OLDER. THE RISK FOR DOWNS SYNDROME INCREASES WITH ADVANCING MATERNAL AGE. FOR WOMEN 35 YEARS OF AGE OR OLDER, GENETIC COUNSELING AND CONSIDERATION OF AMNIOCENTESIS ARE RECOMMENDED, REGARDLESS OF MSAFP TEST RESULTS.

ELEVATED MATERNAL SERUM ALPHA-FETOPROTEIN (MSAFP) VALUES INDICATE AN INCREASED RISK FOR OPEN NEURAL TUBE DEFECTS (NTD), SUCH AS ANENCEPHALY AND SPINA BIFIDA. FOLLOW-UP TESTING SHOULD BE CONSIDERED FOR WOMEN WHOSE RISK FOR OPEN NEURAL TUBE DEFECTS (NTD) EXCEEDS THE GENERAL POPULATION RISK OF 1 IN 500 (1 IN 900 FOR BLACKS). MSAFP CONCENTRATIONS WITHIN THE NORMAL RANGE REDUCE THE LIKELIHOOD OF THESE DEFECTS, BUT CANNOT EXCLUDE ALL ABNORMALITIES.

MSAFP REFERENCE RANGE
0.5 - 2.0 MOM
(0.5 - 1.4 MOM FOR INSULIN-DEPENDENT DIABETICS)
FOR DOWN SYNDROME, THE LOWER CUTOFF MAY VARY
WITH PATIENT'S AGE; SEE "MSAFP RISK DOWN SYND"

GESTATIONAL AGE (WEEKS)	MEDIAN NG/ML
14	25.6
15	29.9
16	34.8
17	40.6
18	47.3
19	55.1
20	64.3
21	74.9

>> END OF REPORT <<

S

T

S
T
Stacek, Theresa Acct. # TS8504 Dr. Bennata

Theresa Starch

4/30 age 21 LMP 4/15 28 days / flow 4 days - mod flow $\bar{c}$ pregnancy $\bar{c}$ abortion B/P 94/60
UTI as child mono 79 Retroverted uterus 1/88.
Pelvic + leg pain x 8 yrs. (R) pelvic swelling
Family history - ↑BP. stroke, diabetes.
Physical + Pap - Chest - N Thyroid - N Ad. - N
Extremities - N Vulva - N Vagina N Ovaries - tender
Nordette 28
Poss Endometriosis - Nordette 28 Evaluation booklet.

7/11 age 22
heavy bleeding $\bar{c}$ last menses x 7 days
LMP 6/30 cramping + ↓ BA Contra - 0

Stevens, Sam M.D.
St. Patrick Tower, Ste. 450
Payneville, TX 77777

The Pathology Laboratory
A Professional Medical Corporation

LABORATORY REPORT

PATIENT NAME	PATIENT ID	ROOM NO.	AGE	SEX	REFERRING PHYSICIAN
STACEK, THERESA	TS8504		21	F	BENNATA

PAGE	REQUISITION NO.	ACCESSION NO.	LAB REF.#	COLLECTION DATE & TIME	LOG-IN-DATE	REPORT DATE	& TIME
1	4013599X	903512L		4-15		4-17	8:13

OB PANEL

TYPE & RH: O POSITIVE
ANTIBODY SCREEN: NONE DETECTED

RPR: NON-REACTIVE
RUBELLA TITER: IMMUNE
HBSAG: NEGATIVE
HIV: NEGATIVE

CBC

WBC	4.2x	10^3
RBC	4.26x	10^6
HGB	13.3	g/dl
HCT	38.7	%
MCV	90.8	um
MCH	31.2	pg
MCHC	34.4	g/dl
RDW	12.8	%
PLT	200.x	10^3

DIFFERENTIAL

SEG	75
BAND	5
LYMPH	19
MONO	1
EOSIN	
BASO	
ATYP LYMPH	
META	

COMMENTS:

URINALYSIS

COLOR	YELLOW
CHARACTER	SL. HAZY
SP. GRAVITY	1.015
pH	7.5
PROTEIN	NEG
GLUCOSE	NEG
ACETONE	NEG
BILE	NEG
OCC. BLOOD	NEG
NITRITE	NEG
UROBILINOGEN	0.2

WBC/HPF	OCCASIONAL
RBC/HPF	0-1
CASTS/LPF	
EPITH	FEW
BACTERIA	1+
CRYSTALS	
PARASITES	
MUCUS	LIGHT
YEAST	

COMMENTS:

DATE: 4-19

TECH: ____________

Stevens, Sam M.D.
St. Patrick Tower, Ste. 450
Payneville, TX 77777

The Pathology Laboratory
A Professional Medical Corporation

LABORATORY REPORT

PATIENT NAME	PATIENT ID	ROOM NO.	AGE	SEX	REFERRING PHYSICIAN
STACEK, THERESA	TS8504		21	F	BENNATA

PAGE	REQUISITION NO.	ACCESSION NO.	LAB REF. #	COLLECTION DATE & TIME	LOG-IN-DATE	REPORT DATE	& TIME
1	4012579X	902122L		05/01	05/01		11:25

CYTOLOGY REPORT: CYTOPATHOLOGY (CERVICAL SMEAR)

CLINICAL HISTORY: TO BE COMPLETED BY REFERRING PHYSICIAN

SPECIMEN SOURCE: ☑ CERVIX ☐ VCE ☐ ENDOCERVIX ☐ VAGINA ☐ OTHER

LMP 4/5 PARA GRAV Age first pregnancy

PRIOR PAP CLASS (circle) None I II III IV IV V DATE

☐ Pregnant
☐ Postpartum
☐ Post Abortion
☐ Post Menop
☐ Hysterectomy
☐ Recent Cautery
☐ Susp. Lesion
☐ Prior CA _______
☐ Others ________________________________

☐ Spotting
☐ Discharge
☐ Ectropion
☐ IUD
☐ BC Pills
☐ Hormone Rx
☐ Condyloma
☐ Herpes

	Normal	Abnormal
Lugol's	☐	☐
Colpo	☐	☐
Cx Bx	☐	☐
Cx Cone	☐	☐
D & C	☐	☐

MATURATION INDEX
☐ Marked Estrogen effect (more than 60% superficial cells)
☐ Moderate Estrogen Effect (25 % to 60% superficial cells)
☑ Slight Estrogen Effect (up to 25% superficial cells)
☐ No evident Estrogen Effect (more than 25% intermediate cells & no superficial cells)
☐ Atrophic Smear (more than 75% parabasal cells)

Cells Present:
☐ White blood cells
☐ Mixed bacteria
☐ B. Vaginalis
☐ Endometrials

☐ Red blood cells
☐ Fungus
☐ Histiocytes
☑ Endocervicals (NO)

☐ Trichomonads
☐ G. Vaginalis (Clue Cell)
☐ Others ________________

DIAGNOSIS:

___✓___ CLASS I — NO EVIDENCE OF DYSPLASIA OR MALIGNANCY
_______ CLASS II — BENIGN ATYPIAS
☐ Reactive or inflammatory atypia
☐ Atypical squamous metaplasia
☐ Reparative atypia
☐ Condyloma
☐ Herpes

_______ CLASS III — DYSPLASIAS
☐ Mild Dysplasia (CIN I)
☐ Moderate Dysplasia (CIN II)

_______ CLASS IV — SEVERE DYSPLASIA/CARCINOMA IN SITU (CIN III)
_______ CLASS V — CARCINOMAS
_______ CLASS O — SMEAR UNSUITABLE FOR EVALUATION

COMMENTS:

CLINICAL PATHOLOGIST	DATE REPORTED	ROOM	ACCESSION NO.

Initial Pregnancy Profile

Date: mo / day / yr 4/14

HOLLISTER maternal/newborn RECORD SYSTEM

PATIENT IDENTIFICATION

Patient's name: Theresa Stacek

History Since LMP (✓) Check and detail all positive findings below. Use reference numbers.

1. Headaches ☑ c̄ nausea
2. Nausea/vomiting ☑ better last 2 wks
3. Abdominal pain ☑ cramping (occasional) U/S pain @ umbilicus (Hx of)
4. Urinary complaints ☐
5. Vaginal discharge ☑ white
6. Vaginal bleeding ☐
7. Edema (specify area) ☐
8. Febrile episode ☐
9. Rubella exposure ☐
10. Other viral exposure ☐
11. Radiation exposure ☐
12. ______ ☐
13. ______ ☐
14. Contraception prior to conception None ☒

Type ______

Last used mo / day / yr ______

15. Nutritional Assessment

☐ Adequate ☐ Inadequate

☒ Nutritional counseling

Remarks: Milk products

16. Medications Since LMP

☐ None ☐ Exposure to drugs

Describe: ______

Initial Physical Examination Height ☐ Weight ☐ Pregravid weight ☐ B.P. ☐ / Pulse ☐ OPTIONAL

SYSTEM	Normal	Abn	Check and detail all abnormal findings below. Use reference numbers.
17. Skin	☑	☐	
18. EENT	☑	☐	
19. Mouth	☑	☐	
20. Neck	☑	☐	Supple
21. Chest	☑	☐	clear
22. Breast	☑	☐	s̄ mass
23. Heart	☑	☐	RR c̄ murmer
24. Lungs	☑	☐	clear
25. Abdomen	☑	☐	soft
26. Musculoskeletal	☑	☐	
27. Extremities	☑	☐	
28. Neurologic	☑	☐	
Pelvic Examination			
29. Ext. genitalia	☑	☐	
30. Vagina	☑	☐	
31. Cervix	☑	☐	
32. Uterus (describe)	☑	☐	4/19 11/wks
33. Adnexa	☐	☐	
34. Rectum	☐	☐	
35. Other	☐	☐	

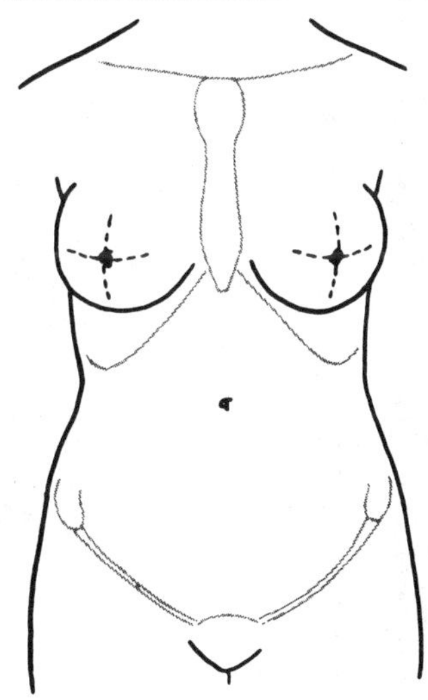

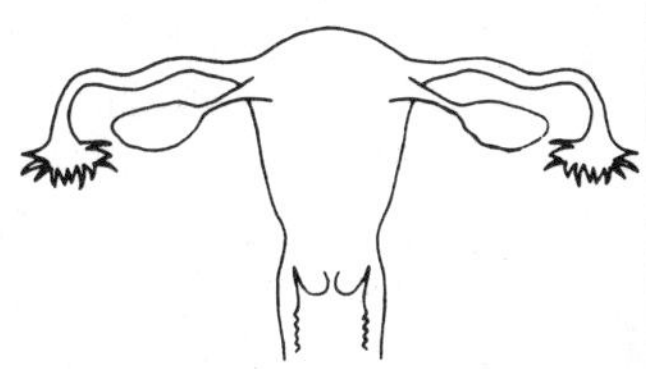

Bony Pelvis

36 Diag. conj. ______ 37 Shape sacrum ______ 38 S.S. notch ______ 39 Ischial spines ______

40 Pubic arch ______ 41 Trans. outlet ______ 42 Post sag. diam. ______ 43 Coccyx ______

44. Classification ☐ Gynecoid ☐ Android ☐ Anthropoid ☐ Platypelloid

45. Estimation ☐ Adequate ☐ Borderline ☐ Contracted

Exam done on mo / day / yr ______ by:

Patient Information

PLEASE PRINT

PATIENT NAME Theresa Stacek AGE 21

ADDRESS 421 Southwood BIRTHDATE 6/15

Payneville, Tx 77777 SEX F

SOCIAL SECURITY 777-22-3333 MARITAL STATUS M PHONE (713) 573-7397

EMPLOYER MedBooks PHONE (800) 443-7397

Please complete if patient is a minor or another party will be responsible for bill.

RESPONSIBLE PARTY ______ RELATION ______

ADDRESS (IF DIFFERENT) ______

SOCIAL SECURITY ______ BIRTHDATE ______ PHONE ( ) ______

TYPE OF COVERAGE: MEDICARE MEDICAID (GROUP) SELF PAY OTHER

MEDICARE ______ PART A PART B

NAME ON CARD MEDICARE NUMBER

MEDICAID ______

NAME ON CARD MEDICAID NUMBER EFFECTIVE DATE

PRIMARY HEALTH INSURANCE BlueCross / Blue Sheild of Texas

COMPANY NAME ADDRESS

Robert Stacek 324RS6789

POLICY HOLDER POLICY NUMBER GROUP NUMBER

SECONDARY HEALTH INSURANCE ______

COMPANY NAME ADDRESS

POLICY HOLDER POLICY NUMBER GROUP NUMBER

I REQUEST THAT PAYMENT OF AUTHORIZED INSURANCE BENEFITS BE MADE EITHER TO ME OR ON MY BEHALF TO THE UNDERSIGNED PROVIDER FOR SERVICES FURNISHED ME BY THAT PHYSICIAN. I PERMIT A COPY OF THIS AUTHORIZATION TO BE USED IN PLACE OF MY ORIGINAL SIGNATURE AND AUTHORIZE ANY HOLDER OF MEDICAL INFORMATION ABOUT ME TO RELEASE TO THE HEALTH CARE FINANCING ADMINISTRATION OR ITS AGENTS ANY INFORMATION NEEDED TO DETERMINE THESE BENEFITS OR THE BENEFITS PAYABLE FOR RELATED SERVICES.

Theresa Stacek 4/30

PATIENT/GUARDIAN SIGNATURE DATE

Prenatal Flow Record

HOLLISTER
maternal/newborn
RECORD SYSTEM

PATIENT IDENTIFICATION

Patient's name: Theresa Stacek

Historical Risk Factors and Assessment

- [0] Has no known risk
- [1] Is "at risk"
- [2] Is at **high risk**

Continuing Risk Assessment Guide (revise RISK STATUS)

Date	At risk factors	Date	**High risk** factors
/	Uterine/cervical malformation	/	Diabetes mellitus
/	Suspect pelvis	/	Hypertension
/	Rh negative (nonsensitized)	/	Thrombophlebitis
/	Anemia (Hct <30%:Hgb <10%)	/	Herpes (type 2)
/	Venereal disease	/	Rh sensitization
/	Acute pyelonephritis	/	Uterine bleeding
/	Failure to gain weight	/	Hydramnios
/	Abnormal presentation	/	Severe preeclampsia
/	Postterm pregnancy	/	Fetal growth retardation
/	Alcohol use	/	Premature rupt. membranes
/		/	Multiple pregnancy (preterm)
/		/	Alcohol and drug abuse
/		/	
/		/	

Initial Prenatal Screen	Date: mo/day/yr	Additional Lab Findings: Test	Date	Result	Date	Result
Hct/Hgb	38.7/13.3	Hct/Hgb	10/11	37.8/12.7	/	
Patient's Blood type and Rh	O+	Blood sugar	/		/	
Antibody	ND	Antibody	/		/	
Serology	NR		/		/	
Rubella titer	Immune	Bacteriuria	/		/	
Urinalysis micro	✓		/		/	
Pap test	I	Herpes	/	Neg	/	
Cervical culture	Neg	Strep	10/15	Neg	/	
HBSAE	Neg	HIV	/	Neg	/	

LMP mo/day/yr: 2/3 | EDC mo/day/yr: 11/10 | Quickening date mo/day/yr:

Medication Sensitivity ☐ None known or:

- ☐ Initial prenatal instructions
- ☐ Attends prenatal classes
- ☐ Do herpes culture
- ☐ Do antenatal RhoGam
- ☐ For sterilization
- ☐ Circumcision
- ☐ Needs rubella vaccine
- ☐ Breast ☐ Bottle feeding

Amniocentesis
Explained on mo / day
☐ Accepted ☐ Rejected by patient

VBAC or C-Section
☐ OR records reviewed
Explained on mo / day
☐ Candidate for VBAC
☐ For Cesarean section

G: II | T: | Pt: | A: I | L:

Age: 22

Pre-gravid: 1

Baby's physician:

Visit date 19__	Weight this visit	Blood pressure	Urine protein	Urine Sugar	Est. weeks gestation (dates/size)	Fundal height	Fetal heart rate/quadrant	Edema			RISK STATUS (0,1,2)	Notes	Return visit	Sig
4/19	123	102/60	-	-	10½/10½	11 wks	+	-	F	c vits		strep GC + pap ? about Unisom denies hx herpes nausea + vomiting	1 mo	[illegible]
/		/			/		+					[illegible] bid	1 mo	[illegible]
5/19	(120)	122/84	tr	-	14/14	15 wks	⊕ 148	-				cramping on + off ↓ BA still vomiting on + off Cx closed	1	[illegible]
(6/2)	c/o severe sharp pains to left side, back [illegible] getting more intense > TO OB													[illegible]
6/22	126	104/80	tr	-	18/18	20	⊕ 136	-				achy feeling in ovary area tightening feeling	1 mo	[illegible]
7/23	132	98/70	tr	-	/	21	⊕ 130	-				movements slowed down u/s c/o B/[illegible]		[illegible]
8/31	139½	110/60	tr	-	/	25	⊕ 140					Fe vit [illegible]	TM	
9/28	145	98/74	tr	-	34/34	31	⊕ 138	-				Fe vits [illegible]	2 wks	
10/11	152	120/74	tr	-	35/35	34	⊕	—				Fe vits strep, herpes, hgb [illegible]	1 wk	[illegible]
10/18	155	118/60	-	-	36/36	35	⊕ [illegible]					Fe vits	1 wk	[illegible]
10/25	158	124/94	tr	-	/	36	⊕ 140	✓				[illegible]		[illegible]
11/3	164	112/80	tr	[illegible]	39/39	37	⊕ [illegible]					Fe vits hot flashes [illegible]	1 wk	[illegible]
/		/			/		+							

Physician's signature

Labor and Delivery Summary

HOLLISTER® maternal/newborn RECORD SYSTEM

51324

Stacek, Theresa #22
Bennata, Darby #7004
9/12/70

Labor Summary

G	T	Pt	A	L	Type and Rh
2			1	1	

Presentation — **Position**: POP

- ☐ Vertex
- ☒ Face or brow
- ☐ Breech ______
- ☐ Transverse lie ☐ Compound
- ☐ Unknown

Intrapartum Events ☐ None

- ☐ No prenatal care
- ☐ Preterm labor (≤ 37 wks.)
- ☐ Postterm (≥ 42 wks.)
- ☐ Febrile (≥ 100.4°)
- ☐ PROM (≥ 1 hr. before onset of labor)
- ☐ Meconium
- ☐ Foul smelling fluid
- ☐ Hydramnios
- ☐ Abruption
- ☐ Placenta previa
- ☐ Bleeding-site undetermined
- ☐ Toxemia (mild) (severe)
- ☐ Seizure activity
- ☐ Precipitous labor (< 3 hrs.)
- ☐ Prolonged labor (≥ 20 hrs.)
- ☐ Prolonged latent phase
- ☐ Prolonged active phase
- ☐ Prolonged 2nd stage (> 2.5 hrs.)
- ☐ Secondary arrest of dilatation
- ☐ Cephalopelvic disproportion
- ☐ Cord prolapse
- ☐ Decreased FHT variability
- ☐ Extended fetal bradycardia
- ☐ Extended fetal tachycardia
- ☐ Multiple late decelerations
- ☐ Multiple variable decelerations
- ☐ Acidosis (pH < 7.2)
- ☐ Anesthetic complications
- ☒ POP to Face presentation
- ☐ ______

Induction ☐ None
☐ ARM ☐ Oxytoc. ☐ ______

Augmentation ☐ None
☒ ARM ☒ Oxytoc. ☐ ______

Monitor ☐ None

	FHT	UC
External	☒	☒
Internal	☐	☐

Medications — Total dosage

- Demerol 50mg
- Phen 25mg IM

Time of last narcotic ______ A/P

Delivery Data

Method of Delivery

Cephalic
- ☐ Spontaneous — Type
- ☐ Low forceps
- ☐ Mid forceps ______
- ☐ Rotation ______ to ______
- ☐ Vacuum extraction

Breech
- ☐ Spontaneous
- ☐ Partial extraction (assisted)
- ☐ Total extraction
- ☐ Forceps to A.C. head

Cesarean (details in operating notes)
- ☒ Low cervical: transverse
- ☐ Low cervical: vertical
- ☐ Classical
- ☐ Cesarean hysterectomy

Placenta
- ☐ Spontaneous
- ☐ Expressed
- ☒ Manual
- ☐ Adherent
- ☐ Ut. exploration

Blood loss: ☐ < 500 ml. ☐ ≥ 500 ml. Specify amount, detail in Remarks (______ ml.)

Configuration
- ☐ Normal
- ☐ Abn. ______

If weighed: ______ gms.

Cord
- ☐ Nuchal cord x ______
- ☐ True knot
- ② ③ Umbilical vessels (3 circled)

Cord blood: (to lab) (refrig.) (discard)
For: ☐ Type & Rh ☒ Coombs ☐ VDRL ☐

Episiotomy ☒ None — Suture
- ☐ Median
- ☐ Mediolateral ______
- ☐ Other ______

Laceration ☒ None
- ① ② ③ ④ Degree perineal
- ☐ Vaginal
- ☐ Cervical
- ☐ Uterine rupture
- ☒ Other ______

Surgical Procedures ☐ None
- ☐ Tubal ligation ☐ Curettage
- ☐ Other See Peri op. record

Delivery Data (cont.)

Delivery Anesthesia ☐ None

1 = Local 2 = Pudendal 3 = Paracervical 4 = Epidural 5 = Spinal 6 = General

No.	Agent/Drug	Dose
6	See Anesthesia notes	

Administered by: Thompson CRNA

Delivery Room Meds. ☐ None

Agent/Drug	Dose	Route	Time	Sig.
Pitocin	20 u.	IV	1830	Thompson CRNA

Chronology

	Date (mo/day/yr)	Time
EDC	11/10	
Admit to hospital	11/4	11:00
Membranes ruptured	11/5	13:40
Onset of labor	11/5	8 AM
Complete cervical dil	11/5	16:00
Delivery of infant	11/5	18:29
Delivery of placenta	11/5	18:30

Infant Data

Apgar Scores

	Heart rate	Respiration	Muscle tone	Reflex irritation	Skin color	Totals
1 min	2	2	2	2	0	8
5 min	2	2	2	2	1	9

Resuscitation ☐ None (spontaneous respiration)
- ☒ Oxygen
- ☐ Bag and mask
- ☐ Intubation
- ☐ Ext. cardiac massage
- ☒ Other Bulb syringe

______ mins. to sustained respiration

Infant Data (cont.)

Medications ☒ None
- ☐ Volume expander
- ☐ Sodium bicarbonate
- ☐ Drug antagonists
- ☐ Umbilical catheter
- ☐ Other ______

Medications checked below were administered in the delivery room. Otherwise reference the Newborn Flow Record.
- ☒ Erythromycin ½%
- ☐ $AgNO_3$ 1% or
- ☒ Aqueous Vitamin K IM

Admin. by: See Nsy MAR

Initial Newborn Exam
- ☐ No observed abnormalities
- ☐ Gross congenital anomalies
- ☐ Mec. staining ☐ Trauma
- ☐ Petechiae ☒ Other

Describe: Edema to face & lips, eyes & nose. Cords received per A LeMat MD — clear

Basic Data

ID bracelet no. 83501
Hospital record no. 51324
☐ Male ☐ Female
Birth order: 1 of ① ② ③ ④
Weight 6-14
Length 18¾

Output
- ☐ Urine
- ☐ Meconium
- ☐ Gastric ______ (ml.)

Transferred:
- ☒ To newborn nursery
- ☐ With mother
- ☐ To NICU
- ☐ ______

Deceased:
- ☐ Antepartum
- ☐ Intrapartum
- ☐ Neonatal (in delivery room)

Date 11/5 — Time 18:40

Remarks: Sterile prep & drape in usual fashion for C/S. Delivered viable female. Father present in delivery. Carried N/B to Nsy c̄ C. Carrier in attendance.

Pediatrician/Resuscitator: A. LeMat MD
Nurse: F. Lowell RN
Assisting: J. Perkins
Attending: D. Bannata
Date completed: 11/5

REPORT OF OPERATION

WEST
CAL-CAM
HOSPITAL

NAME: STACEK, THERESA
DATE: 11-7
SURGEON: LOGAN
ASSISTANT: DARBY BENNATA, M.D.
LEE ALABANTO, M.D.

PREOPERATIVE DIAGNOSIS: LACERATION OF THE BLADDER

POSTOPERATIVE DIAGNOSIS: SAME

OPERATION PERFORMED: BILATERAL DOUBLE PIGTAIL STENT INSERTION WITH REPAIR OF BLADDER LACERATION AND INNER POSITION OF THE PERITONEAL FLAP

ANESTHESIA: ENDOTRACHEAL GENERAL

SUMMARY:

A cesarean section had been performed by Dr. Bennata and a urological assistance requested for an inadvertent bladder laceration.

Inspection of the bladder revealed a T-shaped laceration on the posterior aspect of the bladder with the vertical limb of the T approximately 20 degrees to the right of midline extending from the interureteric ridge, adjacent to the right orifice, obliquely towards the midline for an approximate 4 to 5 cm. distance. The horizontal limb of the laceration then extended approximately 5 cm. possibly 6 cm. in distance. The margins of the laceration were relatively sharp, i.e., jagged indentations were not present. The blood supply was intact to all margins with minimal fulguration required for adequate hemostasis of the margins. For those reasons, it was decided not to incise any of the existing margins.

Indigo carmine was given and efflux seen from both ureteral orifices. To ensure the integrity of the ureters, bilateral 7 French Kwart double pigtail stents were inserted over guide wires with minimal difficulty. Reviewing the laceration, the broader base flap was to the left of midline, however, the base of the flap to the right of midline was approximately 3 to 3.5 cm. and again provided adequate blood supply towards the horizontal limb of the T so that the tip of the flap was not excised.

After placement of the double "J" stent closure was started on the vertical limb with a through and through 2-0 chromic placed at the posterior apex and remained and held for the second layer. Closely spaced through and through 2-0 chromic sutures were then place with all knots on the outside of the bladder. On reaching the anterior end of the vertical limb of the T, the second layer was accomplished with a running inverting 2-0 chromic. The interrupted layer was then placed horizontally in a similar through and through fashion with all knots on the exterior. Two to three sutures were removed from the horizontal layer to extract a gauze sponge from the bladder and the closure of the horizontal layer completed with a second layer of running inverting layer of 2-0 chromic.

The peritoneum was then mobilized from the area adjacent to the posterior wall of the bladder and a broad base flap of peritoneum sutured to the anterior aspect of the lower uterine segment with 3-0 chromic. The flap was then layered out over the anterior vaginal wall interposing this between the suture line on the vertical limb of the T and the uterine and vaginal sutures. Selected sutures ligatures were used for hemastasis prior to placing the peritoneal flap.

Irrigation and closure were then performed by Dr. Bennata. Subsequently, the patient was prepped and draped in a sterile fashion in the supine position, the flexible cystoscope inserted without distending the bladder, but identifying the fact that both "J" stents remained in proper position and no major clots were seen within the bladder. A 22 French Foley catheter was then inserted and placed to close drainage with blood tinged urine obtained. The patient was sent to Recovery in satisfactory condition, received no whole blood and pressure remained stable.

Perry Logan, M.D.

cc: Dr. Bennata
dd: 11-4
dt: 11-5
skc

WEST
CAL-CAM
HOSPITAL

RADIOLOGY REPORT

NAME: Stacek, Theresa X-RAY#: 55672 RADIOLOGIST #: 4892
AGE: 22 SEX: F ROOM NO: OP DATE: 3-18
EXAMINATION: OB/US ATTENDING DR: Bennata PATIENT #: TS8504

OB ULTRASOUND:
The study was performed using transvaginal technique. A single fetus is identified with crown rump length of approximately 7.4 mm. This corresponds to the gestational age of 6.7 weeks + or - 0.4 weeks. The estimated date of confinement is November 7. Cardiac activity was identified. The patient's LMP was February 3, which gives a clinically EDC of Nov. 10. The ultrasound and clinical EDC's are in good agreement.

IMPRESSION:
No significant abnormality demonstrated.

RAE/mr
dt: 3-18

Ray Enohose, M.D.

Stevens, Sam M.D.
St. Patrick Tower, Ste. 450
Payneville, TX 77777

The Pathology Laboratory
A Professional Medical Corporation

LABORATORY REPORT

PATIENT NAME	PATIENT ID	ROOM NO.	AGE	SEX	PHYSICIAN
STACEK, THERESA	TS8504		22	F	BENNATA

PAGE	REQUISITION NO.	ACCESSION NO.	LAB REF.#	COLLECTION DATE & TIME	LOG-IN-DATE	REPORT DATE	& TIME
1	4026579X	912652L	LA 70634	04/19		04-19	4:06

CYTOLOGY REPORT: CYTOPATHOLOGY (CERVICAL SMEAR)

CLINICAL HISTORY: TO BE COMPLETED BY REFERRING PHYSICIAN

SPECIMEN SOURCE: ☒ CERVIX ☐ VCE ☐ ENDOCERVIX ☐ VAGINA ☐ OTHER

LMP 2/3 PARA GRAV Age first pregnancy

PRIOR PAP CLASS (circle) None I II III IV IV V DATE

☒ Pregnant
☐ Postpartum
☐ Post Abortion
☐ Post Menop
☐ Hysterectomy
☐ Recent Cautery
☐ Susp. Lesion
☐ Prior CA _______
☐ Others _______

☐ Spotting
☐ Discharge
☐ Ectropion
☐ IUD
☐ BC Pills
☐ Hormone Rx
☐ Condyloma
☐ Herpes

	Normal	Abnormal
Lugol's	☐	☐
Colpo	☐	☐
Cx Bx	☐	☐
Cx Cone	☐	☐
D & C	☐	☐

MATURATION INDEX
☐ Marked Estrogen effect (more than 60% superficial cells)
☐ Moderate Estrogen Effect (25 % to 60% superficial cells)
☐ Slight Estrogen Effect (up to 25% superficial cells)
☐ No evident Estrogen Effect (more than 25% intermediate cells & no superficial cells)
☐ Atrophic Smear (more than 75% parabasal cells)

Cells Present:
☐ White blood cells
☐ Mixed bacteria
☐ B. Vaginalis
☐ Endometrials
☐ Red blood cells
☐ Fungus
☐ Histiocytes
☐ Endocervicals
☐ Trichomonads
☐ G. Vaginalis (Clue Cell)
☐ Others _______

DIAGNOSIS:

✓ CLASS I — NO EVIDENCE OF DYSPLASIA OR MALIGNANCY
_______ CLASS II — BENIGN ATYPIAS
☐ Reactive or inflammatory atypia
☐ Atypical squamous metaplasia
☐ Reparative atypia
☐ Condyloma
☐ Herpes

_______ CLASS III — DYSPLASIAS
☐ Mild Dysplasia (CIN I)
☐ Moderate Dysplasia (CIN II)

_______ CLASS IV — SEVERE DYSPLASIA/CARCINOMA IN SITU (CIN III)
_______ CLASS V — CARCINOMAS
_______ CLASS O — SMEAR UNSUITABLE FOR EVALUATION

COMMENTS:

CLINICAL PATHOLOGIST	DATE REPORTED	ROOM	ACCESSION NO.

WEST
CAL-CAM
HOSPITAL

RADIOLOGY REPORT

NAME: Stacek, Theresa X-RAY#: 55682 RADIOLOGIST #: 19780
AGE: 22 SEX: F ROOM NO: OP DATE: 7-26
EXAMINATION: OB U/S ATTENDING DR: Bennata PATIENT #: TS8504

OB ULTRASOUND
A single fetus was identified in vertex presentation. Fetal movement and heartbeat were identified. The heart rate was 139 beats per minute. The placenta is located in the fundus and is Grade I. The amount of amniotic fluid appears to be within normal limits.

Gestational age was estimated from measurement of the biparietal diameter, head, circumference, abdominal circumference, and femoral length. These were 62, 137, 207, and 46 mm, respectively, suggesting gestational ages of 25.3, 25.7, 25.2 and 25.4 weeks, respectively. Overall gestational age is estimated at 25.1 +/- 1.8 weeks with the EDC November 8.

BWJ/tmg
dd: 7-26
dt: 7-26
dsrp: 7-26

Bryan W. James, M.D.

RADIOLOGY REPORT

WEST
CAL-CAM
HOSPITAL

NAME: Stacek, Theresa	X-RAY#:	55671	RADIOLOGIST #:	18937
AGE: 22 SEX: F	ROOM NO:	OP	DATE:	10-26
EXAMINATION: BE	ATTENDING DR:	Bennata	PATIENT #:	TS8504

BARIUM ENEMA:
The sigmoid colon is redundant. The cecum is within the pelvis near the midline and projects over the sigmoid colon on the overhead films. No reflux was seen into the terminal ileum. There are no fixed filling defects seen to suggest a polyp. No diverticula are identified. The appendix is partially visualized within the pelvis on the postevac film.

IMPRESSION:
No significant abnormality demonstrated. The cecum and appendix is located in the mid aspect of the pelvis near the midline. In this location, appendicitis could present as pelvic pain.

RAD/mr
dt: 10-26

Ray Davies, M.D.

WEST
CAL-CAM
HOSPITAL

RADIOLOGY REPORT

NAME:	Stacek, Theresa	X-RAY#:	55671	RADIOLOGIST #:	4892
AGE: 22	SEX: F	ROOM NO:	OP	DATE:	10-27
EXAMINATION:	UGI	ATTENDING DR:	Bennata	PATIENT #:	TS8504

UPPER GI WITH SMALL BOWEL EXAM:
The patient did not find the oral contrast very palatable. The esophagus was not well evaluated since it was not well distended as a result. No ulcer or gastric outlet obstruction is seen. No significant small bowel dilatation is identified. Contrast reached the colon by approximately one hour. Artifact overlies the right upper quadrant on the last delayed film.

IMPRESSION:
No significant abnormality demonstrated.

RAE/mr
dt: 10-27

Ray Enohose, M.D.

WEST CAL-CAM HOSPITAL

REPORT OF OPERATION

NAME: STACEK, THERESA
DATE: 11-7
SURGEON: BENNATA
ASSISTANT: NONE
PREOPERATIVE DIAGNOSIS: IMPACTED FACE PRESENTATION WITH SECONDARY ARREST OF LABOR
POSTOPERATIVE DIAGNOSIS: SAME
OPERATION PERFORMED:
1. PRIMARY LOW TRANSVERSE CESAREAN SECTION WITH INADVERTENT BLADDER ENTRY
2. BLADDER CLOSURE WITH BILATERAL URETERAL STENT PLACEMENT
3. REPAIR OF BLADDER LACERATION
4. FLEXIBLE CYSTOSCOPY

ANESTHESIA: ENDOTRACHEAL GENERAL

The patient is a primigravida with face presentation. Secondary arrest of labor has occurred, and the face has become edematous. Cesarean section has been discussed with the patient's husband and family due to the secondary arrest of labor with face presentation. After consents were signed, the patient was brought to the Operating Room. She was prepped with Betadine scrubs followed by Betadine solution.

General anesthesia was administered by the nurse anesthetist at the patient's request. After successive endotracheal intubation and verification, a Pfannenstiel incision was made and sharp dissection was carried down to the fascia which was identified and split. The peritoneum was identified and incised. The uterus was noted to be centrally positioned. A bladder flap was developed without difficulty. The lower uterine segment was noted to be very thin. A small uterine incision was made, and fluid obtained was clear. The uterine incision was extended bilaterally by transection. The infant's face was impacted into the pelvis and it was very difficult to interpose a hand over the infant's face. Multiple attempts were made to deliver the infant's head by gentle flexion and elevation and were finally successful with delivery of the head. The infant was bulb suctioned well and taken to the heat cradle for further care after the cord was doubly clamped and cut. Cord blood was drawn with a syringe. The placenta was delivered manually intact. The uterus was inspected for rents, tears, or defects. The endometrial cavity was inspected for membranes and placental fragments, and none were found. The fundal region was noted to be intact. Upon inspection of the lower uterine segment, a defect in the anterior surface of the uterus and the dome of the bladder was readily apparent.

Dr. Logan was paged in the hospital for assistance, and he will dictate the bladder closure separately. The patient's husband was apprised of the bladder injury in the operating room, and he was informed that the surgery would take longer than we had previously discussed. IV antibiotics were ordered. The uterine edges were grasped with Babcock clamps with great care taken to avoid the trigon area. The posterior segment of the dome laceration was identified which extended down the posterior wall of the bladder. Intermittent urine efflux could be seen from ureteral orifices. The first uterine layer was closed after inspection of the bladder by Dr. Logan. Closure was running and locking O chromic suture with re-apposition of the uterine wall. Great care was taken to avoid placing stitches in any area near the bladder or ureters. Good hemostasis ensued.

The second uterine layer was closed with imbricating sutures of O chromic, again, with care taken to avoid trauma to the urological structures. The placement of J stents and bladder closure is dictated separately by Dr. Logan. Following bladder closure, the gutters were gently swept clear of clots and old blood with minimal movement of the uterus and bladder. Lap, sponge, and needle count were correct x 2. Peritoneal closure was carried out with running O chromic sutures. Infiltration of the peritoneal layer with local anesthetic was carried out. The fascia was closed with running Novafil

CONTINUED

WEST CAL-CAM HOSPITAL

REPORT OF OPERATION

NAME: STACEK, THERESA

PAGE 2

CONTINUED

O sutures. This layer was also infiltrated with local anesthetic. Subcutaneous layer was closed with interrupted sutures of OO plain. The skin was closed with 3-0 PDS subcuticular sutures. The wound was dressed. Cystoscopy and Foley reinsertion was performed by Dr. Logan.

The patient was awakened from anesthesia and taken to the Recovery area for further care. The patient's family and husband were then informed in detail of the bladder laceration and the corrective procedures performed by Dr. Logan and myself. The need for J stents, prolonged indwelling catheter, subsequent cystoscopy, and possible other surgery (if bleeding or other complications occur) was discussed with the patient's husband. The possibility of infection was also discussed. The family's questions were answered.

Darby Bennata, M.D.
dd: 11-7
dt: 11-8
mc

Obstetric Discharge Summary

HOLLISTER® maternal/newborn RECORD SYSTEM

51,324
Stacek, Theresa #22
Bennata, Darby MD, #7004
9/12/10

Reasons for admission ☑ **Onset of labor** ☐ Induction of labor ☐ Cesarean section ☐ Observation/evaluation
☐ Spontaneous abortion ☐ Other ______

Comments and Other Diagnoses

Procedures: Prenatal ☐ **None**
☐ Amniocentesis ☐ Toxemia mgmt. ☐ ______
☐ Cerclage ☑ Ultrasound ☐ ______
☐ NST ☐ ______ ☐ ______
☐ CST ☐ ______

Procedures: Intrapartum ☐ **Spontaneous vaginal delivery**
☐ Forceps (Low) (Mid) ☐ Cesarean hysterectomy
☐ Rotation ______ to ______ ☐ Episiotomy: ______
☐ Breech extraction (Partial) (Total) ☐ Uterine exploration
☐ Forceps to A.C. head ☐ Tubal ligation
☑ Cesarean: low cervical, transverse ☐ Curettage
☐ Cesarean: low cervical, vertical ☑ bladder closure
☐ Cesarean: classical ☐ ______

Procedures: Postpartum ☐ **None**
☐ Transfusion ______ ☐ RH_0 (D) Ig
☐ P.P. tubal ligation ☐ Rubella Ig
☐ Curettage ☐ ______
☑ Antibiotics ☐ ______

Complications: Operative and Postpartum ☐ **None**
☐ ____° perineal laceration ☐ Spinal headache
☐ (Vaginal) (Cervical) laceration ☐ P.P. eclampsia
☐ Pelvic infection ☐ Hemorrhage
☐ Urinary infection ☐ Phlebitis
☐ Pulmonary infection ☐ Morbidity (undetermined)
☐ Wound infection ☐ ______
☑ bladder injury & closure ☐ ______

Discharge Diagnoses ☑ **Term pregnancy - delivered**
☐ Amnionitis ☐ Premature labor
☐ Antepartum bleeding ☐ Placenta previa
☐ Failed induction ☐ PROM x ______ hours
☐ False labor - undelivered ☐ Spontaneous abortion
☐ Hyperemesis gravidarum ☐ Toxemia of pregnancy
☐ Incompetent cervix ☑ impacted face
☐ Post-date pregnancy ☐ ______

Discharge Information Discharge date: 11 mo / 12 day / yr at 17:00 AM PM

Hct	Hgb	Date
		mo / day / yr

Activity ☐ **Unrestricted** (or): bed rest; following limitations
Diet ☐ **Routine** (or): reg
Medications ☐ **None** (or): see d/c summary
Instructions ☐ **Routine** (or): see d/c summary
Discharge to ☐ **Home** (or): ______ Follow up in 11/19 wks at: w/ Bennata Signature [signature]

Status ☐ **Well** ☐ Recovery (or): ______

Newborn Data (for physician's reference only) ☐ Female ☐ Male (☐ Circ. ☐ No circ.) Weight ______ Length ______
☐ Home with mother (or): ______ ☐ No complications (or): ______

DISCHARGE ADDENDUM

WEST
CAL-CAM
HOSPITAL

NAME: Stacek, Theresa ADMIT DATE: 11-5 DISCHARGE DATE: 11-12
ATTENDING PHYSICIAN: Darby Bennata, M.D.

The patient is being discharged of Duricef oral suspension 500 mg per teaspoon q 12 hours x 10 days, Librax capsules 1 or 2 PO 2 or 3 times daily for gas, SND suppositories #15 A as needed for bladder spasms rectally, Valium 1 by mouth for bladder spasms, Percoset 1 or 2 PO q 4 hours prn pain, Surfax 2 at bedtime. The patient has been instructed about consuming 1 or 2 cans of Ensure daily and instructed in a balanced diet. She is instructed in hydrogen peroxide wound care.

The patient is instructed to remember to notify Dr. Bennata immediately if she has fever, chills, increasing pain anywhere, increased blood in her urine, or any other health concerns. The patient is instructed to return to the Radiology Department at Cal-Cam Hospital at 7:45 a.m. on 11-19 for a cystogram and a follow-up check with Drs. Logan and Bennata. The patient is given my home and office telephone number and my 24 hour beeper number. The patient is being discharged in the care of Beegard Home Health and arrangements have been made with the director, Johanna Daisy.

The Home Health Department has been instructed to evaluate urine output and color and reminding the patient to take her medications. They are also checking to see if the Foley is draining okay and only if totally necessary to irrigate the Foley with normal saline not to exceed 30 cc and let it drain to gravity. Home Health is also instructed to follow the patient's nutritional evaluation and to instruct the patient to remember to notify Dr. Bennata for any changes in her medical condition.

FINAL DIAGNOSIS: IMPACTED FACE PRESENTATION WITH SECONDARY ARREST OF LABOR

OPERATIVE PROCEDURES: PRIMARY LOW TRANSVERSE CESAREAN SECTION WITH INADVERTENT BLADDER ENTRY
BLADDER CLOSURE WITH BILATERAL URETERAL STENT PLACEMENT
REPAIR OF BLADDER LACERATION
FLEXIBLE CYSTOSCOPY

D. Bennata

Darby Bennata, M.D.
dd: 11-12
dt: 11-13
mc

SHORT STAY ADMISSION

WEST
CAL-CAM
HOSPITAL

NAME: STACEK, THERESA ADMIT DATE: 11-14 DISCHARGE DATE: 11-14

ROS:

GENERAL:	No chills, fever, night sweats.
HEENT:	No tinnitus, diplopia, epistaxis.
CARDIORESPIRATORY:	Denies chest pain, PND or DOE.
GI:	No nausea, vomiting, diarrhea, or melena.
GU:	See present illness.
NM:	Noncontributory.

PHYSICAL EXAMINATION:

VITAL SIGNS:	BP; PULSE; RESP; TEMP;
GENERAL:	The patient is an alert, oriented female in no acute distress.
HEENT:	Normocephalic, PERRLA, EOM's intact, fundi benign.
CHEST:	Clear to auscultation and percussion, no rales, rubs or rhonchi. Good symmetry, good inspiratory effort.
HEART:	Regular rhythm without murmur, gallop, click or rub. S1 and S2 within normal limits. PMI left fifth intercostal space in midclavicular line.
BREASTS:	The patient has engorged and extremely tender breasts with no evidence of abscess. She shows no skin changes over her breasts other than erythema.
ABDOMEN:	Soft, bowel sounds normal activity. She has slight right costovertebral angle tenderness and minimal left costophrenic angle tenderness.
EXTREMITIES:	No cyanosis, clubbing or edema. Full range of motion in all joints.
NEUROLOGICAL:	Cranial nerves 2-12 grossly intact. Deep tendon reflexes 2+ out of 3+ and bilaterally equal. No abnormal reflexes are elicited.

PROGRESS: The patient was admitted and given an IV antibiotic dosage and then was discharged to begin oral Phloxine 400 mg. PO q 12 hours at home.

OPERATION: NONE

CONDITION: The patient is eating and ambulating.

DIAGNOSIS: POST PARTUM MASTITIS
STATUS POST PLACEMENT OF J STENTS AND BLADDER REPAIR
POST PARTUM STATUS

Darby Bennata, M.D.
dd: 11-14
dt: 11-15
mc

WEST CAL-CAM HOSPITAL

RADIOLOGY REPORT

NAME: Stacek, Theresa X-RAY#: 55835 RADIOLOGIST #: 19780
AGE: 23 SEX: F ROOM NO: OP DATE: 11-19
EXAMINATION: Cystogram ATTENDING DR: Bennata PATIENT #: TS8504

CYSTOGRAM:
On the scout film, there are some small phleboliths in the lower pelvic region. Bilateral stent catheters are noted in place with the lower ends in the bladder. No significant bony abnormalities are demonstrated.

After insertion of the contrast into the bladder, there appeared to be some filling defects within the bladder which may be either air bubbles or possibly blood clots. There is irregularity of the posterior aspect of the bladder. No extravasation is demonstrated. The right ureter continues to show gross dilatation. Left ureter appears slightly dilated.

BWJ/tmg
dd: 11-19
dt: 11-19
dsrp: 11-19

Bryan W. James, M.D.

REPORT OF OPERATION

WEST
CAL-CAM
HOSPITAL

NAME: STACEK, THERESA
DATE: 11-19
SURGEON: P. LOGAN
ASSISTANT:
PREOPERATIVE DIAGNOSIS: INDWELLING BILATERAL DOUBLE "J" STENTS AND FOLEY CATHETER, STATUS POST BLADDER REPAIR
POSTOPERATIVE DIAGNOSIS: CYSTOGRAM
OPERATION PERFORMED: FLEXIBLE CYSTOSCOPY
REMOVAL OF DOUBLE "J" STENT
ANESTHESIA: I.V. SEDATION

In X-ray and after multiple attempts, an IV access was finally obtained. Approximately 14 - 15 mg. of Valium was given intravenously, slowly, and at intervals during the procedure.

Initially, a Static cystogram was obtained with a maximum instilled volume of 200 ccs. creating a sense of distention and discomfort to the patient. AP, oblique, and lateral views were obtained with a post drainage film, all failing to indicate extravasation. Contrast did fill the upper collecting systems through the double "J" stents. The patient was prepped and draped in a sterile fashion in the frog-leg position. The flexible scope was inserted identifying bullous edema of the suture lines on the posterior bladder wall. The left orifice could not be distinguished as the bullae obscured the view through the double "J" stent could be seen exiting through the bullae on the left trigone. The right orifice could be identified with its double "J" stent exiting. The sutures from the double "J" were secured together and grasping with a biopsy forcep both double "Js" were removed. A 16 Foley catheter was inserted and placed to leg bag drainage and will be removed in four days.

cc: Darby Bennata, M.D.
dd: 11-19
dt: 11-19
jed

Perry Logan, M.D.

S

T

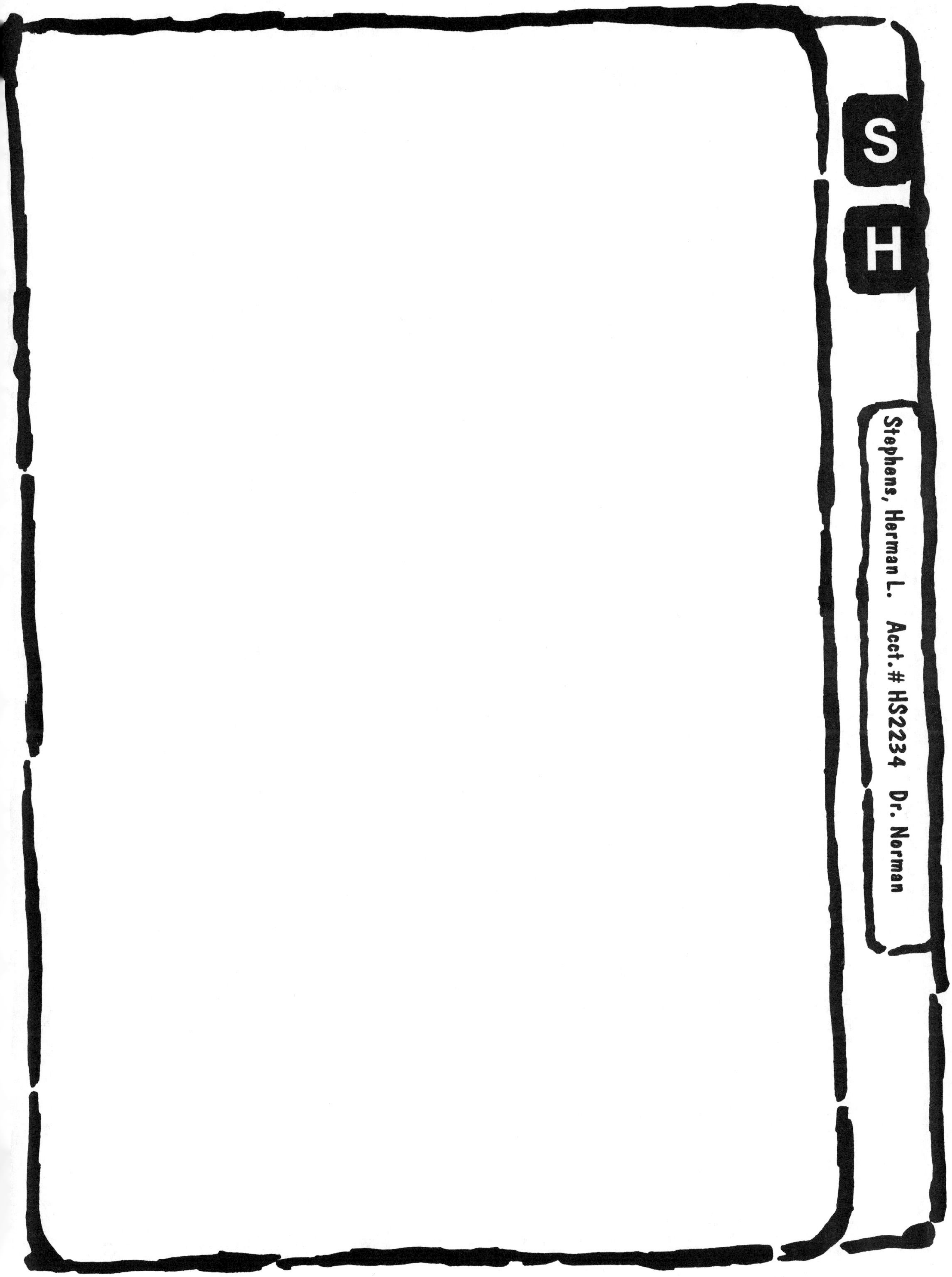
S
H
Stephens, Herman L. Acct. # HS2234 Dr. Norman

Patient Information

PLEASE PRINT

PATIENT NAME Herman L. Stephens AGE 34
ADDRESS 2222 Rose St. BIRTHDATE 2/10
Paynesville, TX 77777 SEX M
SOCIAL SECURITY 001-11-2222 MARITAL STATUS M PHONE (713) 973-7397
EMPLOYER Halliburton PHONE (-)

Please complete if patient is a minor or another party will be responsible for bill.

RESPONSIBLE PARTY Self RELATION
ADDRESS (IF DIFFERENT)
SOCIAL SECURITY BIRTHDATE PHONE ( )

TYPE OF COVERAGE: MEDICARE MEDICAID (GROUP) SELF PAY OTHER

MEDICARE ___ NAME ON CARD ___ MEDICARE NUMBER ___ PART A PART B

MEDICAID ___ NAME ON CARD ___ MEDICAID NUMBER ___ EFFECTIVE DATE

PRIMARY HEALTH INSURANCE
Southwest — COMPANY NAME; — ADDRESS
Herman Stephens — POLICY HOLDER; 001-11-2222 — POLICY NUMBER; B5238 — GROUP NUMBER

SECONDARY HEALTH INSURANCE
COMPANY NAME ADDRESS
POLICY HOLDER POLICY NUMBER GROUP NUMBER

I REQUEST THAT PAYMENT OF AUTHORIZED INSURANCE BENEFITS BE MADE EITHER TO ME OR ON MY BEHALF TO THE UNDERSIGNED PROVIDER FOR SERVICES FURNISHED ME BY THAT PHYSICIAN. I PERMIT A COPY OF THIS AUTHORIZATION TO BE USED IN PLACE OF MY ORIGINAL SIGNATURE AND AUTHORIZE ANY HOLDER OF MEDICAL INFORMATION ABOUT ME TO RELEASE TO THE HEALTH CARE FINANCING ADMINISTRATION OR ITS AGENTS ANY INFORMATION NEEDED TO DETERMINE THESE BENEFITS OR THE BENEFITS PAYABLE FOR RELATED SERVICES.

Herman Stephens — PATIENT/GUARDIAN SIGNATURE 2/6 — DATE

H L. STEPHEN

2/6 4 yr history of back pain. Works

HIST: as a cementer. Does a lot of heavy lifting. Back, a few days ago, gave out as he made a sudden turn while sitting in his truck. Minutes later on bending down it again caught. He describes the pain as a sharp pain across the low back, especially in the RT. No hist. of leg Radiation. Bending over agg's pain while sitting up helps.

H. L. Stephen

2/6 cont'd PX Back

There are no sensory changes

All musculature good and equal bilaterally including the extensor hallucis longus.

True leg lengths 36 7/8 bilat.

Circumferential measurements

6" ↓ patella 15 1/2 bilat.

X Rays: L-Spine Series : Early L5-S1 disc degeneration

DX: Early deg disc disease

Rx: T-4

B-30 (T T.i.d / i T.i.d) > c̄ meals

Flex 10 mgms

Soaks

Williams flexion exercises

Off slip 2/6 to 2/18

Ret 2/16

H. L. STEPHEN

2/6 cont'd

PX

Back

Paraspinous muscle spasm is mild

Sciatic Nerve compression is negative

Active Motion: flexion: finger tips to toes, no pain

extension 30° with some pain at L3-4 levels

RT & LT lat bending: finger tips to knees bilaterally, no pain

Rt & Lt Rotation: 75° bilaterally, no pain

Pelvic compression and/or distraction → negative

Hips: no abnormalities noted

Straight leg raising: 75° bilaterally, no pain. Dorsi flexion of the feet does not agg. nor cause sciatic Nerve Radiation

K J's & A J's are brisk & equal bilat.

H. L. STEPHEN
2/6 cont'd

PX:
BACK

The patient walks without a limp.
He undresses cautiously with apparent difficulty and discomfort
There is no external evidence of injury
There is a mild Lt. dorsal and a Rt. lumbar scoliosis with the apices at D5 & L2 respectively
The normal lumbar lordosis is well preserved

H.L. STEPHEN

2/11 Phone Call – No better!

℞ – Continue present Regime

Obtain C.T. lumbar spine

at ST Pat's

2/12 CT L-Spine: Disc herniation

L5-S1

℞ – Will refer to DR Litel

Re second opinion

2/19 DR Litel feels pt has no

Radiculopathy & is progressing

satisfactorily. To continue present

Regime. Ret prn.

Paul Litel, M.D.
Professional Corporation
Neurosurgery
780 Ryan Street
Payneville, Texas 77777

February 19

Dr. M. Norman
651 South Ryan Street
Payneville, Texas 77777

RE: H. Stephens

Dear Mark:

I saw Herman in the office on February 18. As you will recall that on about February 6, he injured his back. He reached into the icebox to get a coke and had a sudden pain. Thereafter, he had pain in his back and into his right leg. The leg discomfort is not particularly severe and in fact it is much less than it has been in the past. He has had some numbness. The major complaint in his leg now however, is some numbness that goes down the back of his thigh. The examination is not remarkable. I find no neurologic findings. The cat scan shows a herniated disk at L5 S1 in the left side.

It is my impression that he has some symptoms to suggest radiculopathy but he has improved significantly and at this time is really fairly comfortable. I told him to continue his conservative activities and if he should worsen, to let me see him. I believe however, he will do well. I appreciate very much the opportunity to see this interesting patient.

Sincerely,

Paul Litel

Paul Litel, M.D.

PL/ps

RADIOLOGY

St. Patrick Hospital
Payneville, Texas 77777

NAME: Herman L. Stephens
REQUESTED BY: Dr. M. Norman
AGE: 25
ROOM #: n/a **DATE:** 2/12

PROCEDURE PERFORMED:

CT Lumbar Spine

Serial 3mm sections were obtained from the lower aspect of L3 through S1. The L3-4 disc appears normal. At L4-5, there is mild circumferential bulging of the disc without evidence of herniation. At L5-6, there is a left sided paramedian herniation of the disc with displacement of the left nerve root and epidural fat planes.

No other definite abnormalities are identified.

IMPRESSION:

1. LEFT PARAMEDIAN DISC HERNIATION AT L5-S1
2. MILD DISC BULGING AT L4-5

SAGITTAL RECONSTRUCTION: This reveals no additional findings. The neural foramen appear normally bilateral.

R.N. Brown, M.D./pms

T

S

Thompson, Sandy Acct.# ST4233 Dr. Thomas

Patient Information

PLEASE PRINT

PATIENT NAME Sandy Thompson AGE 23

ADDRESS 455 E. Third St. NE BIRTHDATE 8-18

Paynesville TX 77777 SEX F

SOCIAL SECURITY 666-22-3333 MARITAL STATUS S PHONE (713) 973-7397

EMPLOYER Burger Palace PHONE ( )

Please complete if patient is a minor or another party will be responsible for bill.

RESPONSIBLE PARTY Bill Thompson RELATION Father

ADDRESS (IF DIFFERENT) same

SOCIAL SECURITY 666-33-4444 BIRTHDATE 11-1-42 PHONE (713) 973-7397

TYPE OF COVERAGE: MEDICARE MEDICAID (GROUP) SELF PAY (OTHER)

MEDICARE ______ PART A PART B

NAME ON CARD / MEDICARE NUMBER

MEDICAID ______

NAME ON CARD / MEDICAID NUMBER / EFFECTIVE DATE

PRIMARY HEALTH INSURANCE

Travellers

COMPANY NAME / ADDRESS

Bill Thompson 666-33-4444 3TS471

POLICY HOLDER / POLICY NUMBER / GROUP NUMBER

SECONDARY HEALTH INSURANCE

BC/BS of Texas

COMPANY NAME / ADDRESS

Norma Thompson 666443333 —

POLICY HOLDER / POLICY NUMBER / GROUP NUMBER

I REQUEST THAT PAYMENT OF AUTHORIZED INSURANCE BENEFITS BE MADE EITHER TO ME OR ON MY BEHALF TO THE UNDERSIGNED PROVIDER FOR SERVICES FURNISHED ME BY THAT PHYSICIAN. I PERMIT A COPY OF THIS AUTHORIZATION TO BE USED IN PLACE OF MY ORIGINAL SIGNATURE AND AUTHORIZE ANY HOLDER OF MEDICAL INFORMATION ABOUT ME TO RELEASE TO THE HEALTH CARE FINANCING ADMINISTRATION OR ITS AGENTS ANY INFORMATION NEEDED TO DETERMINE THESE BENEFITS OR THE BENEFITS PAYABLE FOR RELATED SERVICES.

Bill Thompson 12-2

PATIENT/GUARDIAN SIGNATURE DATE

S. Thompson
12-2

20 y/o WF burned Ⓡ hand 2 days ago c̄ hot grease while @ work. Seen @ St. Patrick ER + tx c̄ bid silvadene + sterile dsg. Referred for F/U.

PE: 1° burns dorsal web spaces Ⓡ hand; no blistering no signs of ischemia or infection; minimal edema.

Imp: 1° burns Ⓡ hand.

Recc: 1) cont. silvadene bid + sterile dsg.
2) elevate Ⓡ hand.
3) RTC Mon.

H Thomas MD

12-6

Wounds have healed nicely s̄ scarring. D/C dsg. + silvadene. RTC 2wks.

H Thomas MD

T

S

W
A
Whitmore, Albert Acct. # AW3456 Dr. Thomas

Patient Information

PLEASE PRINT

PATIENT NAME ALBERT Whitmore AGE 34

ADDRESS 123 ABNEY STReet BIRTHDATE 1/1/1

PAYNEVILLE, TX. 77777 SEX M

SOCIAL SECURITY 345-67-8901 MARITAL STATUS M PHONE (713) 973-7397

EMPLOYER ______ PHONE (800) 443-7397

Please complete if patient is a minor or another party will be responsible for bill.

RESPONSIBLE PARTY SELF RELATION ______

ADDRESS (IF DIFFERENT) ______

SOCIAL SECURITY ______ BIRTHDATE ______ PHONE ( ) ______

TYPE OF COVERAGE: MEDICARE MEDICAID GROUP SELF PAY OTHER

MEDICARE ______ PART A PART B

NAME ON CARD MEDICARE NUMBER

MEDICAID ______

NAME ON CARD MEDICAID NUMBER EFFECTIVE DATE

PRIMARY HEALTH INSURANCE EQUITABLE P.O. BOX 65000 DALLAS, TX. 75565-5464

COMPANY NAME ADDRESS

ALBERT Whitmore AW 555-444 MB-222333

POLICY HOLDER POLICY NUMBER GROUP NUMBER

SECONDARY HEALTH INSURANCE ______

COMPANY NAME ADDRESS

______

POLICY HOLDER POLICY NUMBER GROUP NUMBER

I REQUEST THAT PAYMENT OF AUTHORIZED INSURANCE BENEFITS BE MADE EITHER TO ME OR ON MY BEHALF TO THE UNDERSIGNED PROVIDER FOR SERVICES FURNISHED ME BY THAT PHYSICIAN. I PERMIT A COPY OF THIS AUTHORIZATION TO BE USED IN PLACE OF MY ORIGINAL SIGNATURE AND AUTHORIZE ANY HOLDER OF MEDICAL INFORMATION ABOUT ME TO RELEASE TO THE HEALTH CARE FINANCING ADMINISTRATION OR ITS AGENTS ANY INFORMATION NEEDED TO DETERMINE THESE BENEFITS OR THE BENEFITS PAYABLE FOR RELATED SERVICES.

Albert Whitmore Oct. '29

PATIENT/GUARDIAN SIGNATURE DATE

10-29 Albert Whitmore

34 y/o M sustained blunt trauma to nose on volleyball pole 3 days ago. Pt. has noted a change in the shape of his nose + difficulty breathing on the Ⓡ. Seen in ER after accident. X-Ray revealed fx both nasal bones c̄ displacement. PMH – ∅ Meds – "pain pills from ER". NKA

PE: moderate edema nasal dorsum small laceration repaired – healing well deviation of nasal vault into Ⓡ septal deviation into Ⓡ c̄ AW obstruction – no septal hematoma

Imp: nasal fx c̄ displacement + septal deviation.

10-29 cont'd

Recc – closed nasal/septal reduction under anesth. Procedure explained in detail c̄ pt. including risks, complications + alternate procedures. Explained to pt. that closed reduction is not always successful + that he may need further reconstructive surgery.

H C Thomas MD

10/31 A. Whitmore

1 days s/p closed reduction nasal fx + septal dislocation. Pt c̄ c/o nausea yesterday. Packing removed splint intact – Nasal vault appears in midline. RTC 1 wk for splint removal.

H C Thomas MD

11/6 A. Whitmore

Splint removed, nasal vault in midline; moderate edema (R > L). RTC ī mo. Avoid all nasal trauma.

H Thomas MD

12/4

N/S

12/11

6 wks. S/P closed nasal/septal reduction. No c/o breathing difficulty @ this time. Nasal vault still c̄ significant amt. of deviation.

H Thomas MD

X-RAY CONSULTATION

St. Patrick Hospital

Payneville, Texas 77777

Name:	Albert Whitmore	**Age:**	34		
Requested By:	Dr. Thomas	**Room #:**	ER	**Date:**	Oct. 30

Examination: Nasal fracture

Diagnosis: 3 view X-rays reveal fracture of both nasal bones with displacement and displacement of the septum.

X-Ray # 81-4239

R.R. John, M.D./ch

Radiologist

REPORT OF OPERATION

St. Patrick Hospital
Payneville, Texas 77777

Case #: AW3456

Name: Albert Whitmore | **Date:** Oct. 30 | **Room #:** 235

Surgeon: Dr. H. Thomas | **Assistant:** None

Anesthetist: Dr. Maywood | **Started:** | **Ended:**

Preoperative Diagnosis: Nasal fracture with septal dislocation.

Postoperative Diagnosis: Same

Operation: Closed reduction of nasal fracture
Closed reduction of septal dislocation

INDICATIONS: The patient was referred to my office after being seen several days ago in the Emergency Room following blunt trauma to his nose. At the time of examination in the Emergency Room, X-rays revealed fracture of both nasal bones with displacement and displacement of the septum.

On physician examination, these findings were noted. The patient had gross deviation of the nasal vault of the right as well as septal deviation to the right. It was elected to attempt a closed reduction of the septal deviation and nasal bone fracture. The patient understands that he may still need reconstructive nasal surgery in the future.

PROCEDURE: The patient was placed on the operating room table in the supine position. After intubation, the nares were inspected with a nasal speculum. The septum was indeed noted to be deviated to the right and dislocated caudally. The Asch forceps were inserted and the septum was reduced into the midline. Attention was then turned toward the bony nasal vault. A knife hand was inserted under the left nasal bone which was fractured and depressed with upward and outward pressure. The left nasal bone was reduced. Manual pressure on the right nasal bone medially also achieved reduction here. The nasal bones were then molded in the midline. 1/2 inch Vaseline packing was used in each of the nares. A nasal splint was then applied. The patient tolerated the procedure well.

DR. H. Thomas/md
CC:
DICT: Oct. 30
TRAN: Oct 31

PLEASE DO NOT STAPLE IN THIS AREA

APPROVED OMB-0938-0008

PICA

HEALTH INSURANCE CLAIM FORM

PICA

1. MEDICARE (Medicare #) MEDICAID (Medicaid #) CHAMPUS (Sponsor's SSN) CHAMPVA (VA File #) GROUP HEALTH PLAN (SSN or ID) FECA BLK LUNG (SSN) OTHER (ID)

1a. INSURED'S I.D. NUMBER (FOR PROGRAM IN ITEM 1)

2. PATIENT'S NAME (Last Name, First Name, Middle Initial)

3. PATIENT'S BIRTH DATE MM | DD | YY SEX M F

4. INSURED'S NAME (Last Name, First Name, Middle Initial)

5. PATIENT'S ADDRESS (No., Street)

6. PATIENT RELATIONSHIP TO INSURED Self Spouse Child Other

7. INSURED'S ADDRESS (No., Street)

CITY STATE

8. PATIENT STATUS Single Married Other

CITY STATE

ZIP CODE TELEPHONE (Include Area Code) ( )

Employed Full-Time Student Part-Time Student

ZIP CODE TELEPHONE (INCLUDE AREA CODE) ( )

9. OTHER INSURED'S NAME (Last Name, First Name, Middle Initial)

10. IS PATIENT'S CONDITION RELATED TO:

11. INSURED'S POLICY GROUP OR FECA NUMBER

a. OTHER INSURED'S POLICY OR GROUP NUMBER

a. EMPLOYMENT? (CURRENT OR PREVIOUS) YES NO

a. INSURED'S DATE OF BIRTH MM | DD | YY SEX M F

b. OTHER INSURED'S DATE OF BIRTH MM | DD | YY SEX M F

b. AUTO ACCIDENT? YES NO PLACE (State)

b. EMPLOYER'S NAME OR SCHOOL NAME

c. EMPLOYER'S NAME OR SCHOOL NAME

c. OTHER ACCIDENT? YES NO

c. INSURANCE PLAN NAME OR PROGRAM NAME

d. INSURANCE PLAN NAME OR PROGRAM NAME

10d. RESERVED FOR LOCAL USE

d. IS THERE ANOTHER HEALTH BENEFIT PLAN? YES NO ***If yes,*** return to and complete item 9 a-d.

READ BACK OF FORM BEFORE COMPLETING & SIGNING THIS FORM.

12. PATIENT'S OR AUTHORIZED PERSON'S SIGNATURE I authorize the release of any medical or other information necessary to process this claim. I also request payment of government benefits either to myself or to the party who accepts assignment below.

SIGNED ______________ DATE ______________

13. INSURED'S OR AUTHORIZED PERSON'S SIGNATURE I authorize payment of medical benefits to the undersigned physician or supplier for services described below.

SIGNED ______________

14. DATE OF CURRENT: MM | DD | YY ◀ ILLNESS (First symptom) OR INJURY (Accident) OR PREGNANCY(LMP)

15. IF PATIENT HAS HAD SAME OR SIMILAR ILLNESS. GIVE FIRST DATE MM | DD | YY

16. DATES PATIENT UNABLE TO WORK IN CURRENT OCCUPATION FROM MM | DD | YY TO MM | DD | YY

17. NAME OF REFERRING PHYSICIAN OR OTHER SOURCE

17a. I.D. NUMBER OF REFERRING PHYSICIAN

18. HOSPITALIZATION DATES RELATED TO CURRENT SERVICES FROM MM | DD | YY TO MM | DD | YY

19. RESERVED FOR LOCAL USE

20. OUTSIDE LAB? YES NO $ CHARGES

21. DIAGNOSIS OR NATURE OF ILLNESS OR INJURY. (RELATE ITEMS 1,2,3 OR 4 TO ITEM 24E BY LINE)

1. ___ . __
2. ___ . __
3. ___ . __
4. ___ . __

22. MEDICAID RESUBMISSION CODE ORIGINAL REF. NO.

23. PRIOR AUTHORIZATION NUMBER

24. A DATE(S) OF SERVICE From MM DD YY	To MM DD YY	B Place of Service	C Type of Service	D PROCEDURES, SERVICES, OR SUPPLIES (Explain Unusual Circumstances) CPT/HCPCS | MODIFIER	E DIAGNOSIS CODE	F $ CHARGES	G DAYS OR UNITS	H EPSDT Family Plan	I EMG	J COB	K RESERVED FOR LOCAL USE
1											
2											
3											
4											
5											
6											

25. FEDERAL TAX I.D. NUMBER SSN EIN

26. PATIENT'S ACCOUNT NO.

27. ACCEPT ASSIGNMENT? (For govt. claims, see back) YES NO

28. TOTAL CHARGE $

29. AMOUNT PAID $

30. BALANCE DUE $

31. SIGNATURE OF PHYSICIAN OR SUPPLIER INCLUDING DEGREES OR CREDENTIALS (I certify that the statements on the reverse apply to this bill and are made a part thereof.)

SIGNED DATE

32. NAME AND ADDRESS OF FACILITY WHERE SERVICES WERE RENDERED (If other than home or office)

33. PHYSICIAN'S, SUPPLIER'S BILLING NAME, ADDRESS, ZIP CODE & PHONE #

PIN# GRP#

(APPROVED BY AMA COUNCIL ON MEDICAL SERVICE 8/88)

PLEASE PRINT OR TYPE

FORM HCFA-1500 (12-90), FORM RRB-1500, FORM OWCP-1500

PLEASE
DO NOT
STAPLE
IN THIS
AREA

APPROVED OMB-0938-0008

PICA

HEALTH INSURANCE CLAIM FORM

PICA

1. MEDICARE (Medicare #) MEDICAID (Medicaid #) CHAMPUS (Sponsor's SSN) CHAMPVA (VA File #) GROUP HEALTH PLAN (SSN or ID) FECA BLK LUNG (SSN) OTHER (ID)

1a. INSURED'S I.D. NUMBER (FOR PROGRAM IN ITEM 1)

2. PATIENT'S NAME (Last Name, First Name, Middle Initial)

3. PATIENT'S BIRTH DATE MM DD YY SEX M F

4. INSURED'S NAME (Last Name, First Name, Middle Initial)

5. PATIENT'S ADDRESS (No., Street)

6. PATIENT RELATIONSHIP TO INSURED Self Spouse Child Other

7. INSURED'S ADDRESS (No., Street)

CITY STATE

8. PATIENT STATUS Single Married Other

CITY STATE

ZIP CODE TELEPHONE (Include Area Code) ( )

Employed Full-Time Student Part-Time Student

ZIP CODE TELEPHONE (INCLUDE AREA CODE) ( )

9. OTHER INSURED'S NAME (Last Name, First Name, Middle Initial)

10. IS PATIENT'S CONDITION RELATED TO:

11. INSURED'S POLICY GROUP OR FECA NUMBER

a. OTHER INSURED'S POLICY OR GROUP NUMBER

a. EMPLOYMENT? (CURRENT OR PREVIOUS) YES NO

a. INSURED'S DATE OF BIRTH MM DD YY SEX M F

b. OTHER INSURED'S DATE OF BIRTH MM DD YY SEX M F

b. AUTO ACCIDENT? PLACE (State) YES NO

b. EMPLOYER'S NAME OR SCHOOL NAME

c. EMPLOYER'S NAME OR SCHOOL NAME

c. OTHER ACCIDENT? YES NO

c. INSURANCE PLAN NAME OR PROGRAM NAME

d. INSURANCE PLAN NAME OR PROGRAM NAME

10d. RESERVED FOR LOCAL USE

d. IS THERE ANOTHER HEALTH BENEFIT PLAN? YES NO *If yes*, return to and complete item 9 a-d.

READ BACK OF FORM BEFORE COMPLETING & SIGNING THIS FORM.

12. PATIENT'S OR AUTHORIZED PERSON'S SIGNATURE I authorize the release of any medical or other information necessary to process this claim. I also request payment of government benefits either to myself or to the party who accepts assignment below.

SIGNED ____________ DATE ____________

13. INSURED'S OR AUTHORIZED PERSON'S SIGNATURE I authorize payment of medical benefits to the undersigned physician or supplier for services described below.

SIGNED ____________

14. DATE OF CURRENT: MM DD YY ILLNESS (First symptom) OR INJURY (Accident) OR PREGNANCY(LMP)

15. IF PATIENT HAS HAD SAME OR SIMILAR ILLNESS. GIVE FIRST DATE MM DD YY

16. DATES PATIENT UNABLE TO WORK IN CURRENT OCCUPATION FROM MM DD YY TO MM DD YY

17. NAME OF REFERRING PHYSICIAN OR OTHER SOURCE

17a. I.D. NUMBER OF REFERRING PHYSICIAN

18. HOSPITALIZATION DATES RELATED TO CURRENT SERVICES FROM MM DD YY TO MM DD YY

19. RESERVED FOR LOCAL USE

20. OUTSIDE LAB? YES NO $ CHARGES

21. DIAGNOSIS OR NATURE OF ILLNESS OR INJURY. (RELATE ITEMS 1,2,3 OR 4 TO ITEM 24E BY LINE)

1. ____ . __
2. ____ . __
3. ____ . __
4. ____ . __

22. MEDICAID RESUBMISSION CODE ORIGINAL REF. NO.

23. PRIOR AUTHORIZATION NUMBER

24. A DATE(S) OF SERVICE From MM DD YY	To MM DD YY	B Place of Service	C Type of Service	D PROCEDURES, SERVICES, OR SUPPLIES (Explain Unusual Circumstances) CPT/HCPCS MODIFIER	E DIAGNOSIS CODE	F $ CHARGES	G DAYS OR UNITS	H EPSDT Family Plan	I EMG	J COB	K RESERVED FOR LOCAL USE
1											
2											
3											
4											
5											
6											

25. FEDERAL TAX I.D. NUMBER SSN EIN

26. PATIENT'S ACCOUNT NO.

27. ACCEPT ASSIGNMENT? (For govt. claims, see back) YES NO

28. TOTAL CHARGE $

29. AMOUNT PAID $

30. BALANCE DUE $

31. SIGNATURE OF PHYSICIAN OR SUPPLIER INCLUDING DEGREES OR CREDENTIALS (I certify that the statements on the reverse apply to this bill and are made a part thereof.)

SIGNED DATE

32. NAME AND ADDRESS OF FACILITY WHERE SERVICES WERE RENDERED (If other than home or office)

33. PHYSICIAN'S, SUPPLIER'S BILLING NAME, ADDRESS, ZIP CODE & PHONE #

PIN# GRP#

(APPROVED BY AMA COUNCIL ON MEDICAL SERVICE 8/88)

PLEASE PRINT OR TYPE

FORM HCFA-1500 (12-90), FORM RRB-1500, FORM OWCP-1500

PLEASE DO NOT STAPLE IN THIS AREA

APPROVED OMB-0938-0008

PICA

HEALTH INSURANCE CLAIM FORM

PICA

1. MEDICARE (Medicare #) | MEDICAID (Medicaid #) | CHAMPUS (Sponsor's SSN) | CHAMPVA (VA File #) | GROUP HEALTH PLAN (SSN or ID) | FECA BLK LUNG (SSN) | OTHER (ID)

1a. INSURED'S I.D. NUMBER (FOR PROGRAM IN ITEM 1)

2. PATIENT'S NAME (Last Name, First Name, Middle Initial)

3. PATIENT'S BIRTH DATE MM | DD | YY — SEX M F

4. INSURED'S NAME (Last Name, First Name, Middle Initial)

5. PATIENT'S ADDRESS (No., Street)

6. PATIENT RELATIONSHIP TO INSURED — Self Spouse Child Other

7. INSURED'S ADDRESS (No., Street)

CITY — STATE

8. PATIENT STATUS — Single Married Other — Employed Full-Time Student Part-Time Student

CITY — STATE

ZIP CODE — TELEPHONE (Include Area Code) ( )

ZIP CODE — TELEPHONE (INCLUDE AREA CODE) ( )

9. OTHER INSURED'S NAME (Last Name, First Name, Middle Initial)

10. IS PATIENT'S CONDITION RELATED TO:

11. INSURED'S POLICY GROUP OR FECA NUMBER

a. OTHER INSURED'S POLICY OR GROUP NUMBER

a. EMPLOYMENT? (CURRENT OR PREVIOUS) YES NO

a. INSURED'S DATE OF BIRTH MM | DD | YY — SEX M F

b. OTHER INSURED'S DATE OF BIRTH MM | DD | YY — SEX M F

b. AUTO ACCIDENT? YES NO — PLACE (State)

b. EMPLOYER'S NAME OR SCHOOL NAME

c. EMPLOYER'S NAME OR SCHOOL NAME

c. OTHER ACCIDENT? YES NO

c. INSURANCE PLAN NAME OR PROGRAM NAME

d. INSURANCE PLAN NAME OR PROGRAM NAME

10d. RESERVED FOR LOCAL USE

d. IS THERE ANOTHER HEALTH BENEFIT PLAN? YES NO *If yes*, return to and complete item 9 a-d.

READ BACK OF FORM BEFORE COMPLETING & SIGNING THIS FORM.

12. PATIENT'S OR AUTHORIZED PERSON'S SIGNATURE I authorize the release of any medical or other information necessary to process this claim. I also request payment of government benefits either to myself or to the party who accepts assignment below.

SIGNED ____ DATE ____

13. INSURED'S OR AUTHORIZED PERSON'S SIGNATURE I authorize payment of medical benefits to the undersigned physician or supplier for services described below.

SIGNED ____

14. DATE OF CURRENT: MM | DD | YY — ILLNESS (First symptom) OR INJURY (Accident) OR PREGNANCY(LMP)

15. IF PATIENT HAS HAD SAME OR SIMILAR ILLNESS. GIVE FIRST DATE MM | DD | YY

16. DATES PATIENT UNABLE TO WORK IN CURRENT OCCUPATION FROM MM | DD | YY TO MM | DD | YY

17. NAME OF REFERRING PHYSICIAN OR OTHER SOURCE

17a. I.D. NUMBER OF REFERRING PHYSICIAN

18. HOSPITALIZATION DATES RELATED TO CURRENT SERVICES FROM MM | DD | YY TO MM | DD | YY

19. RESERVED FOR LOCAL USE

20. OUTSIDE LAB? YES NO — $ CHARGES

21. DIAGNOSIS OR NATURE OF ILLNESS OR INJURY. (RELATE ITEMS 1,2,3 OR 4 TO ITEM 24E BY LINE)

1. ____ . __
2. ____ . __
3. ____ . __
4. ____ . __

22. MEDICAID RESUBMISSION CODE — ORIGINAL REF. NO.

23. PRIOR AUTHORIZATION NUMBER

24. A DATE(S) OF SERVICE From MM DD YY To MM DD YY	B Place of Service	C Type of Service	D PROCEDURES, SERVICES, OR SUPPLIES (Explain Unusual Circumstances) CPT/HCPCS | MODIFIER	E DIAGNOSIS CODE	F $ CHARGES	G DAYS OR UNITS	H EPSDT Family Plan	I EMG	J COB	K RESERVED FOR LOCAL USE
1										
2										
3										
4										
5										
6										

25. FEDERAL TAX I.D. NUMBER — SSN EIN

26. PATIENT'S ACCOUNT NO.

27. ACCEPT ASSIGNMENT? (For govt. claims, see back) YES NO

28. TOTAL CHARGE $

29. AMOUNT PAID $

30. BALANCE DUE $

31. SIGNATURE OF PHYSICIAN OR SUPPLIER INCLUDING DEGREES OR CREDENTIALS (I certify that the statements on the reverse apply to this bill and are made a part thereof.)

SIGNED ____ DATE ____

32. NAME AND ADDRESS OF FACILITY WHERE SERVICES WERE RENDERED (If other than home or office)

33. PHYSICIAN'S, SUPPLIER'S BILLING NAME, ADDRESS, ZIP CODE & PHONE #

PIN# — GRP#

(APPROVED BY AMA COUNCIL ON MEDICAL SERVICE 8/88)

PLEASE PRINT OR TYPE

FORM HCFA-1500 (12-90), FORM RRB-1500, FORM OWCP-1500

PLEASE DO NOT STAPLE IN THIS AREA

APPROVED OMB-0938-0008

PICA

HEALTH INSURANCE CLAIM FORM

PICA

1. MEDICARE (Medicare #) MEDICAID (Medicaid #) CHAMPUS (Sponsor's SSN) CHAMPVA (VA File #) GROUP HEALTH PLAN (SSN or ID) FECA BLK LUNG (SSN) OTHER (ID)

1a. INSURED'S I.D. NUMBER (FOR PROGRAM IN ITEM 1)

2. PATIENT'S NAME (Last Name, First Name, Middle Initial)

3. PATIENT'S BIRTH DATE MM DD YY SEX M F

4. INSURED'S NAME (Last Name, First Name, Middle Initial)

5. PATIENT'S ADDRESS (No., Street)

6. PATIENT RELATIONSHIP TO INSURED Self Spouse Child Other

7. INSURED'S ADDRESS (No., Street)

CITY STATE

8. PATIENT STATUS Single Married Other

CITY STATE

ZIP CODE TELEPHONE (Include Area Code) ( )

Employed Full-Time Student Part-Time Student

ZIP CODE TELEPHONE (INCLUDE AREA CODE) ( )

9. OTHER INSURED'S NAME (Last Name, First Name, Middle Initial)

10. IS PATIENT'S CONDITION RELATED TO:

11. INSURED'S POLICY GROUP OR FECA NUMBER

a. OTHER INSURED'S POLICY OR GROUP NUMBER

a. EMPLOYMENT? (CURRENT OR PREVIOUS) YES NO

a. INSURED'S DATE OF BIRTH MM DD YY SEX M F

b. OTHER INSURED'S DATE OF BIRTH MM DD YY SEX M F

b. AUTO ACCIDENT? YES NO PLACE (State)

b. EMPLOYER'S NAME OR SCHOOL NAME

c. EMPLOYER'S NAME OR SCHOOL NAME

c. OTHER ACCIDENT? YES NO

c. INSURANCE PLAN NAME OR PROGRAM NAME

d. INSURANCE PLAN NAME OR PROGRAM NAME

10d. RESERVED FOR LOCAL USE

d. IS THERE ANOTHER HEALTH BENEFIT PLAN? YES NO *If yes*, return to and complete item 9 a-d.

READ BACK OF FORM BEFORE COMPLETING & SIGNING THIS FORM.

12. PATIENT'S OR AUTHORIZED PERSON'S SIGNATURE I authorize the release of any medical or other information necessary to process this claim. I also request payment of government benefits either to myself or to the party who accepts assignment below.

SIGNED ____________________ DATE ____________

13. INSURED'S OR AUTHORIZED PERSON'S SIGNATURE I authorize payment of medical benefits to the undersigned physician or supplier for services described below.

SIGNED ____________________

14. DATE OF CURRENT: MM DD YY ILLNESS (First symptom) OR INJURY (Accident) OR PREGNANCY(LMP)

15. IF PATIENT HAS HAD SAME OR SIMILAR ILLNESS. GIVE FIRST DATE MM DD YY

16. DATES PATIENT UNABLE TO WORK IN CURRENT OCCUPATION FROM MM DD YY TO MM DD YY

17. NAME OF REFERRING PHYSICIAN OR OTHER SOURCE

17a. I.D. NUMBER OF REFERRING PHYSICIAN

18. HOSPITALIZATION DATES RELATED TO CURRENT SERVICES FROM MM DD YY TO MM DD YY

19. RESERVED FOR LOCAL USE

20. OUTSIDE LAB? YES NO $ CHARGES

21. DIAGNOSIS OR NATURE OF ILLNESS OR INJURY. (RELATE ITEMS 1,2,3 OR 4 TO ITEM 24E BY LINE)

1. ____ . __

3. ____ . __

2. ____ . __

4. ____ . __

22. MEDICAID RESUBMISSION CODE ORIGINAL REF. NO.

23. PRIOR AUTHORIZATION NUMBER

24. A DATE(S) OF SERVICE From MM DD YY To MM DD YY	B Place of Service	C Type of Service	D PROCEDURES, SERVICES, OR SUPPLIES (Explain Unusual Circumstances) CPT/HCPCS MODIFIER	E DIAGNOSIS CODE	F $ CHARGES	G DAYS OR UNITS	H EPSDT Family Plan	I EMG	J COB	K RESERVED FOR LOCAL USE
1										
2										
3										
4										
5										
6										

25. FEDERAL TAX I.D. NUMBER SSN EIN

26. PATIENT'S ACCOUNT NO.

27. ACCEPT ASSIGNMENT? (For govt. claims, see back) YES NO

28. TOTAL CHARGE $

29. AMOUNT PAID $

30. BALANCE DUE $

31. SIGNATURE OF PHYSICIAN OR SUPPLIER INCLUDING DEGREES OR CREDENTIALS (I certify that the statements on the reverse apply to this bill and are made a part thereof.)

SIGNED DATE

32. NAME AND ADDRESS OF FACILITY WHERE SERVICES WERE RENDERED (If other than home or office)

33. PHYSICIAN'S, SUPPLIER'S BILLING NAME, ADDRESS, ZIP CODE & PHONE #

PIN# GRP#

(APPROVED BY AMA COUNCIL ON MEDICAL SERVICE 8/88)

PLEASE PRINT OR TYPE

FORM HCFA-1500 (12-90), FORM RRB-1500, FORM OWCP-1500

PLEASE DO NOT STAPLE IN THIS AREA

APPROVED OMB-0938-0008

PICA

HEALTH INSURANCE CLAIM FORM

PICA

1. MEDICARE (Medicare #) | MEDICAID (Medicaid #) | CHAMPUS (Sponsor's SSN) | CHAMPVA (VA File #) | GROUP HEALTH PLAN (SSN or ID) | FECA BLK LUNG (SSN) | OTHER (ID)

1a. INSURED'S I.D. NUMBER (FOR PROGRAM IN ITEM 1)

2. PATIENT'S NAME (Last Name, First Name, Middle Initial)

3. PATIENT'S BIRTH DATE MM DD YY SEX M F

4. INSURED'S NAME (Last Name, First Name, Middle Initial)

5. PATIENT'S ADDRESS (No., Street)

6. PATIENT RELATIONSHIP TO INSURED Self Spouse Child Other

7. INSURED'S ADDRESS (No., Street)

CITY STATE

8. PATIENT STATUS Single Married Other

CITY STATE

ZIP CODE TELEPHONE (Include Area Code) ( )

Employed Full-Time Student Part-Time Student

ZIP CODE TELEPHONE (INCLUDE AREA CODE) ( )

9. OTHER INSURED'S NAME (Last Name, First Name, Middle Initial)

10. IS PATIENT'S CONDITION RELATED TO:

11. INSURED'S POLICY GROUP OR FECA NUMBER

a. OTHER INSURED'S POLICY OR GROUP NUMBER

a. EMPLOYMENT? (CURRENT OR PREVIOUS) YES NO

a. INSURED'S DATE OF BIRTH MM DD YY SEX M F

b. OTHER INSURED'S DATE OF BIRTH MM DD YY SEX M F

b. AUTO ACCIDENT? YES NO PLACE (State)

b. EMPLOYER'S NAME OR SCHOOL NAME

c. EMPLOYER'S NAME OR SCHOOL NAME

c. OTHER ACCIDENT? YES NO

c. INSURANCE PLAN NAME OR PROGRAM NAME

d. INSURANCE PLAN NAME OR PROGRAM NAME

10d. RESERVED FOR LOCAL USE

d. IS THERE ANOTHER HEALTH BENEFIT PLAN? YES NO ***If yes***, return to and complete item 9 a-d.

READ BACK OF FORM BEFORE COMPLETING & SIGNING THIS FORM.

12. PATIENT'S OR AUTHORIZED PERSON'S SIGNATURE I authorize the release of any medical or other information necessary to process this claim. I also request payment of government benefits either to myself or to the party who accepts assignment below.

SIGNED ____________ DATE ____________

13. INSURED'S OR AUTHORIZED PERSON'S SIGNATURE I authorize payment of medical benefits to the undersigned physician or supplier for services described below.

SIGNED ____________

14. DATE OF CURRENT: MM DD YY ILLNESS (First symptom) OR INJURY (Accident) OR PREGNANCY(LMP)

15. IF PATIENT HAS HAD SAME OR SIMILAR ILLNESS. GIVE FIRST DATE MM DD YY

16. DATES PATIENT UNABLE TO WORK IN CURRENT OCCUPATION FROM MM DD YY TO MM DD YY

17. NAME OF REFERRING PHYSICIAN OR OTHER SOURCE

17a. I.D. NUMBER OF REFERRING PHYSICIAN

18. HOSPITALIZATION DATES RELATED TO CURRENT SERVICES FROM MM DD YY TO MM DD YY

19. RESERVED FOR LOCAL USE

20. OUTSIDE LAB? YES NO $ CHARGES

21. DIAGNOSIS OR NATURE OF ILLNESS OR INJURY. (RELATE ITEMS 1,2,3 OR 4 TO ITEM 24E BY LINE)

1. ____ . __

2. ____ . __

3. ____ . __

4. ____ . __

22. MEDICAID RESUBMISSION CODE ORIGINAL REF. NO.

23. PRIOR AUTHORIZATION NUMBER

24.	A					B	C	D		E	F	G	H	I	J	K
	DATE(S) OF SERVICE From MM	DD	YY	To MM	DD	YY	Place of Service	Type of Service	PROCEDURES, SERVICES, OR SUPPLIES (Explain Unusual Circumstances) CPT/HCPCS	MODIFIER	DIAGNOSIS CODE	$ CHARGES	DAYS OR UNITS	EPSDT Family Plan	EMG	COB	RESERVED FOR LOCAL USE
1																	
2																	
3																	
4																	
5																	
6																	

25. FEDERAL TAX I.D. NUMBER SSN EIN

26. PATIENT'S ACCOUNT NO.

27. ACCEPT ASSIGNMENT? (For govt. claims, see back) YES NO

28. TOTAL CHARGE $

29. AMOUNT PAID $

30. BALANCE DUE $

31. SIGNATURE OF PHYSICIAN OR SUPPLIER INCLUDING DEGREES OR CREDENTIALS (I certify that the statements on the reverse apply to this bill and are made a part thereof.)

SIGNED DATE

32. NAME AND ADDRESS OF FACILITY WHERE SERVICES WERE RENDERED (If other than home or office)

33. PHYSICIAN'S, SUPPLIER'S BILLING NAME, ADDRESS, ZIP CODE & PHONE #

PIN# GRP#

(APPROVED BY AMA COUNCIL ON MEDICAL SERVICE 8/88)

PLEASE PRINT OR TYPE

FORM HCFA-1500 (12-90), FORM RRB-1500, FORM OWCP-1500

PLEASE
DO NOT
STAPLE
IN THIS
AREA

APPROVED OMB-0938-0008

PICA

HEALTH INSURANCE CLAIM FORM

PICA

1. MEDICARE ☐ (Medicare #) MEDICAID ☐ (Medicaid #) CHAMPUS ☐ (Sponsor's SSN) CHAMPVA ☐ (VA File #) GROUP HEALTH PLAN ☐ (SSN or ID) FECA BLK LUNG ☐ (SSN) OTHER ☐ (ID)

1a. INSURED'S I.D. NUMBER (FOR PROGRAM IN ITEM 1)

2. PATIENT'S NAME (Last Name, First Name, Middle Initial)

3. PATIENT'S BIRTH DATE MM | DD | YY SEX M ☐ F ☐

4. INSURED'S NAME (Last Name, First Name, Middle Initial)

5. PATIENT'S ADDRESS (No., Street)

6. PATIENT RELATIONSHIP TO INSURED Self ☐ Spouse ☐ Child ☐ Other ☐

7. INSURED'S ADDRESS (No., Street)

CITY STATE

8. PATIENT STATUS Single ☐ Married ☐ Other ☐ Employed ☐ Full-Time Student ☐ Part-Time Student ☐

CITY STATE

ZIP CODE TELEPHONE (Include Area Code) ( )

ZIP CODE TELEPHONE (INCLUDE AREA CODE) ( )

9. OTHER INSURED'S NAME (Last Name, First Name, Middle Initial)

a. OTHER INSURED'S POLICY OR GROUP NUMBER

b. OTHER INSURED'S DATE OF BIRTH MM | DD | YY SEX M ☐ F ☐

c. EMPLOYER'S NAME OR SCHOOL NAME

d. INSURANCE PLAN NAME OR PROGRAM NAME

10. IS PATIENT'S CONDITION RELATED TO:

a. EMPLOYMENT? (CURRENT OR PREVIOUS) ☐ YES ☐ NO

b. AUTO ACCIDENT? ☐ YES ☐ NO PLACE (State)

c. OTHER ACCIDENT? ☐ YES ☐ NO

10d. RESERVED FOR LOCAL USE

11. INSURED'S POLICY GROUP OR FECA NUMBER

a. INSURED'S DATE OF BIRTH MM | DD | YY SEX M ☐ F ☐

b. EMPLOYER'S NAME OR SCHOOL NAME

c. INSURANCE PLAN NAME OR PROGRAM NAME

d. IS THERE ANOTHER HEALTH BENEFIT PLAN? ☐ YES ☐ NO *If yes*, return to and complete item 9 a-d.

READ BACK OF FORM BEFORE COMPLETING & SIGNING THIS FORM.

12. PATIENT'S OR AUTHORIZED PERSON'S SIGNATURE I authorize the release of any medical or other information necessary to process this claim. I also request payment of government benefits either to myself or to the party who accepts assignment below.

SIGNED ____________ DATE ____________

13. INSURED'S OR AUTHORIZED PERSON'S SIGNATURE I authorize payment of medical benefits to the undersigned physician or supplier for services described below.

SIGNED ____________

14. DATE OF CURRENT: MM | DD | YY ◀ ILLNESS (First symptom) OR INJURY (Accident) OR PREGNANCY(LMP)

15. IF PATIENT HAS HAD SAME OR SIMILAR ILLNESS. GIVE FIRST DATE MM | DD | YY

16. DATES PATIENT UNABLE TO WORK IN CURRENT OCCUPATION FROM MM | DD | YY TO MM | DD | YY

17. NAME OF REFERRING PHYSICIAN OR OTHER SOURCE

17a. I.D. NUMBER OF REFERRING PHYSICIAN

18. HOSPITALIZATION DATES RELATED TO CURRENT SERVICES FROM MM | DD | YY TO MM | DD | YY

19. RESERVED FOR LOCAL USE

20. OUTSIDE LAB? ☐ YES ☐ NO $ CHARGES

21. DIAGNOSIS OR NATURE OF ILLNESS OR INJURY. (RELATE ITEMS 1,2,3 OR 4 TO ITEM 24E BY LINE)

1. ____ . __
2. ____ . __
3. ____ . __
4. ____ . __

22. MEDICAID RESUBMISSION CODE ORIGINAL REF. NO.

23. PRIOR AUTHORIZATION NUMBER

24. A DATE(S) OF SERVICE From MM	DD	YY	To MM	DD	YY	B Place of Service	C Type of Service	D PROCEDURES, SERVICES, OR SUPPLIES (Explain Unusual Circumstances) CPT/HCPCS | MODIFIER	E DIAGNOSIS CODE	F $ CHARGES	G DAYS OR UNITS	H EPSDT Family Plan	I EMG	J COB	K RESERVED FOR LOCAL USE
1											
2											
3											
4											
5											
6											

25. FEDERAL TAX I.D. NUMBER SSN EIN ☐ ☐

26. PATIENT'S ACCOUNT NO.

27. ACCEPT ASSIGNMENT? (For govt. claims, see back) ☐ YES ☐ NO

28. TOTAL CHARGE $

29. AMOUNT PAID $

30. BALANCE DUE $

31. SIGNATURE OF PHYSICIAN OR SUPPLIER INCLUDING DEGREES OR CREDENTIALS (I certify that the statements on the reverse apply to this bill and are made a part thereof.)

SIGNED DATE

32. NAME AND ADDRESS OF FACILITY WHERE SERVICES WERE RENDERED (If other than home or office)

33. PHYSICIAN'S, SUPPLIER'S BILLING NAME, ADDRESS, ZIP CODE & PHONE #

PIN# GRP#

(APPROVED BY AMA COUNCIL ON MEDICAL SERVICE 8/88)

PLEASE PRINT OR TYPE

FORM HCFA-1500 (12-90), FORM RRB-1500, FORM OWCP-1500

PLEASE DO NOT STAPLE IN THIS AREA

APPROVED OMB-0938-0008

PICA

HEALTH INSURANCE CLAIM FORM

PICA

1. MEDICARE (Medicare #) MEDICAID (Medicaid #) CHAMPUS (Sponsor's SSN) CHAMPVA (VA File #) GROUP HEALTH PLAN (SSN or ID) FECA BLK LUNG (SSN) OTHER (ID)

1a. INSURED'S I.D. NUMBER (FOR PROGRAM IN ITEM 1)

2. PATIENT'S NAME (Last Name, First Name, Middle Initial)

3. PATIENT'S BIRTH DATE MM DD YY SEX M F

4. INSURED'S NAME (Last Name, First Name, Middle Initial)

5. PATIENT'S ADDRESS (No., Street)

CITY STATE

ZIP CODE TELEPHONE (Include Area Code) ( )

6. PATIENT RELATIONSHIP TO INSURED Self Spouse Child Other

8. PATIENT STATUS Single Married Other

Employed Full-Time Student Part-Time Student

7. INSURED'S ADDRESS (No., Street)

CITY STATE

ZIP CODE TELEPHONE (INCLUDE AREA CODE) ( )

9. OTHER INSURED'S NAME (Last Name, First Name, Middle Initial)

a. OTHER INSURED'S POLICY OR GROUP NUMBER

b. OTHER INSURED'S DATE OF BIRTH MM DD YY SEX M F

c. EMPLOYER'S NAME OR SCHOOL NAME

d. INSURANCE PLAN NAME OR PROGRAM NAME

10. IS PATIENT'S CONDITION RELATED TO:

a. EMPLOYMENT? (CURRENT OR PREVIOUS) YES NO

b. AUTO ACCIDENT? PLACE (State) YES NO

c. OTHER ACCIDENT? YES NO

10d. RESERVED FOR LOCAL USE

11. INSURED'S POLICY GROUP OR FECA NUMBER

a. INSURED'S DATE OF BIRTH MM DD YY SEX M F

b. EMPLOYER'S NAME OR SCHOOL NAME

c. INSURANCE PLAN NAME OR PROGRAM NAME

d. IS THERE ANOTHER HEALTH BENEFIT PLAN? YES NO *If yes*, return to and complete item 9 a-d.

READ BACK OF FORM BEFORE COMPLETING & SIGNING THIS FORM.

12. PATIENT'S OR AUTHORIZED PERSON'S SIGNATURE I authorize the release of any medical or other information necessary to process this claim. I also request payment of government benefits either to myself or to the party who accepts assignment below.

SIGNED ________________ DATE ________________

13. INSURED'S OR AUTHORIZED PERSON'S SIGNATURE I authorize payment of medical benefits to the undersigned physician or supplier for services described below.

SIGNED ________________

14. DATE OF CURRENT: MM DD YY ILLNESS (First symptom) OR INJURY (Accident) OR PREGNANCY(LMP)

15. IF PATIENT HAS HAD SAME OR SIMILAR ILLNESS. GIVE FIRST DATE MM DD YY

16. DATES PATIENT UNABLE TO WORK IN CURRENT OCCUPATION FROM MM DD YY TO MM DD YY

17. NAME OF REFERRING PHYSICIAN OR OTHER SOURCE

17a. I.D. NUMBER OF REFERRING PHYSICIAN

18. HOSPITALIZATION DATES RELATED TO CURRENT SERVICES FROM MM DD YY TO MM DD YY

19. RESERVED FOR LOCAL USE

20. OUTSIDE LAB? YES NO $ CHARGES

21. DIAGNOSIS OR NATURE OF ILLNESS OR INJURY. (RELATE ITEMS 1,2,3 OR 4 TO ITEM 24E BY LINE)

1. ___ . __ 3. ___ . __

2. ___ . __ 4. ___ . __

22. MEDICAID RESUBMISSION CODE ORIGINAL REF. NO.

23. PRIOR AUTHORIZATION NUMBER

24. A DATE(S) OF SERVICE From MM DD YY	To MM DD YY	B Place of Service	C Type of Service	D PROCEDURES, SERVICES, OR SUPPLIES (Explain Unusual Circumstances) CPT/HCPCS | MODIFIER	E DIAGNOSIS CODE	F $ CHARGES	G DAYS OR UNITS	H EPSDT Family Plan	I EMG	J COB	K RESERVED FOR LOCAL USE
1											
2											
3											
4											
5											
6											

25. FEDERAL TAX I.D. NUMBER SSN EIN

26. PATIENT'S ACCOUNT NO.

27. ACCEPT ASSIGNMENT? (For govt. claims, see back) YES NO

28. TOTAL CHARGE $

29. AMOUNT PAID $

30. BALANCE DUE $

31. SIGNATURE OF PHYSICIAN OR SUPPLIER INCLUDING DEGREES OR CREDENTIALS (I certify that the statements on the reverse apply to this bill and are made a part thereof.)

SIGNED DATE

32. NAME AND ADDRESS OF FACILITY WHERE SERVICES WERE RENDERED (If other than home or office)

33. PHYSICIAN'S, SUPPLIER'S BILLING NAME, ADDRESS, ZIP CODE & PHONE #

PIN# GRP#

(APPROVED BY AMA COUNCIL ON MEDICAL SERVICE 8/88)

PLEASE PRINT OR TYPE

FORM HCFA-1500 (12-90), FORM RRB-1500, FORM OWCP-1500

PLEASE
DO NOT
STAPLE
IN THIS
AREA

APPROVED OMB-0938-0008

PICA

HEALTH INSURANCE CLAIM FORM

PICA

1. MEDICARE (Medicare #) MEDICAID (Medicaid #) CHAMPUS (Sponsor's SSN) CHAMPVA (VA File #) GROUP HEALTH PLAN (SSN or ID) FECA BLK LUNG (SSN) OTHER (ID)

1a. INSURED'S I.D. NUMBER (FOR PROGRAM IN ITEM 1)

2. PATIENT'S NAME (Last Name, First Name, Middle Initial)

3. PATIENT'S BIRTH DATE MM DD YY SEX M F

4. INSURED'S NAME (Last Name, First Name, Middle Initial)

5. PATIENT'S ADDRESS (No., Street)

6. PATIENT RELATIONSHIP TO INSURED Self Spouse Child Other

7. INSURED'S ADDRESS (No., Street)

CITY STATE

8. PATIENT STATUS Single Married Other

CITY STATE

ZIP CODE TELEPHONE (Include Area Code) ( )

Employed Full-Time Student Part-Time Student

ZIP CODE TELEPHONE (INCLUDE AREA CODE) ( )

9. OTHER INSURED'S NAME (Last Name, First Name, Middle Initial)

10. IS PATIENT'S CONDITION RELATED TO:

11. INSURED'S POLICY GROUP OR FECA NUMBER

a. OTHER INSURED'S POLICY OR GROUP NUMBER

a. EMPLOYMENT? (CURRENT OR PREVIOUS) YES NO

a. INSURED'S DATE OF BIRTH MM DD YY SEX M F

b. OTHER INSURED'S DATE OF BIRTH MM DD YY SEX M F

b. AUTO ACCIDENT? YES NO PLACE (State)

b. EMPLOYER'S NAME OR SCHOOL NAME

c. EMPLOYER'S NAME OR SCHOOL NAME

c. OTHER ACCIDENT? YES NO

c. INSURANCE PLAN NAME OR PROGRAM NAME

d. INSURANCE PLAN NAME OR PROGRAM NAME

10d. RESERVED FOR LOCAL USE

d. IS THERE ANOTHER HEALTH BENEFIT PLAN? YES NO *If yes*, return to and complete item 9 a-d.

READ BACK OF FORM BEFORE COMPLETING & SIGNING THIS FORM.

12. PATIENT'S OR AUTHORIZED PERSON'S SIGNATURE I authorize the release of any medical or other information necessary to process this claim. I also request payment of government benefits either to myself or to the party who accepts assignment below.

SIGNED ______ DATE ______

13. INSURED'S OR AUTHORIZED PERSON'S SIGNATURE I authorize payment of medical benefits to the undersigned physician or supplier for services described below.

SIGNED ______

14. DATE OF CURRENT: MM DD YY ILLNESS (First symptom) OR INJURY (Accident) OR PREGNANCY(LMP)

15. IF PATIENT HAS HAD SAME OR SIMILAR ILLNESS. GIVE FIRST DATE MM DD YY

16. DATES PATIENT UNABLE TO WORK IN CURRENT OCCUPATION FROM MM DD YY TO MM DD YY

17. NAME OF REFERRING PHYSICIAN OR OTHER SOURCE

17a. I.D. NUMBER OF REFERRING PHYSICIAN

18. HOSPITALIZATION DATES RELATED TO CURRENT SERVICES FROM MM DD YY TO MM DD YY

19. RESERVED FOR LOCAL USE

20. OUTSIDE LAB? YES NO $ CHARGES

21. DIAGNOSIS OR NATURE OF ILLNESS OR INJURY. (RELATE ITEMS 1,2,3 OR 4 TO ITEM 24E BY LINE)

1. ___ . __
2. ___ . __
3. ___ . __
4. ___ . __

22. MEDICAID RESUBMISSION CODE ORIGINAL REF. NO.

23. PRIOR AUTHORIZATION NUMBER

24. A DATE(S) OF SERVICE From MM DD YY To MM DD YY	B Place of Service	C Type of Service	D PROCEDURES, SERVICES, OR SUPPLIES (Explain Unusual Circumstances) CPT/HCPCS MODIFIER	E DIAGNOSIS CODE	F $ CHARGES	G DAYS OR UNITS	H EPSDT Family Plan	I EMG	J COB	K RESERVED FOR LOCAL USE
1										
2										
3										
4										
5										
6										

25. FEDERAL TAX I.D. NUMBER SSN EIN

26. PATIENT'S ACCOUNT NO.

27. ACCEPT ASSIGNMENT? (For govt. claims, see back) YES NO

28. TOTAL CHARGE $

29. AMOUNT PAID $

30. BALANCE DUE $

31. SIGNATURE OF PHYSICIAN OR SUPPLIER INCLUDING DEGREES OR CREDENTIALS (I certify that the statements on the reverse apply to this bill and are made a part thereof.)

SIGNED DATE

32. NAME AND ADDRESS OF FACILITY WHERE SERVICES WERE RENDERED (If other than home or office)

33. PHYSICIAN'S, SUPPLIER'S BILLING NAME, ADDRESS, ZIP CODE & PHONE #

PIN# GRP#

(APPROVED BY AMA COUNCIL ON MEDICAL SERVICE 8/88)

PLEASE PRINT OR TYPE

FORM HCFA-1500 (12-90), FORM RRB-1500, FORM OWCP-1500

APPROVED OMB-0938-0008

PLEASE DO NOT STAPLE IN THIS AREA

PICA

HEALTH INSURANCE CLAIM FORM

PICA

1. MEDICARE (Medicare #) MEDICAID (Medicaid #) CHAMPUS (Sponsor's SSN) CHAMPVA (VA File #) GROUP HEALTH PLAN (SSN or ID) FECA BLK LUNG (SSN) OTHER (ID)

1a. INSURED'S I.D. NUMBER (FOR PROGRAM IN ITEM 1)

2. PATIENT'S NAME (Last Name, First Name, Middle Initial)

3. PATIENT'S BIRTH DATE MM DD YY SEX M F

4. INSURED'S NAME (Last Name, First Name, Middle Initial)

5. PATIENT'S ADDRESS (No., Street)

6. PATIENT RELATIONSHIP TO INSURED Self Spouse Child Other

7. INSURED'S ADDRESS (No., Street)

CITY STATE

8. PATIENT STATUS Single Married Other

CITY STATE

ZIP CODE TELEPHONE (Include Area Code) ( )

Employed Full-Time Student Part-Time Student

ZIP CODE TELEPHONE (INCLUDE AREA CODE) ( )

9. OTHER INSURED'S NAME (Last Name, First Name, Middle Initial)

10. IS PATIENT'S CONDITION RELATED TO:

11. INSURED'S POLICY GROUP OR FECA NUMBER

a. OTHER INSURED'S POLICY OR GROUP NUMBER

a. EMPLOYMENT? (CURRENT OR PREVIOUS) YES NO

a. INSURED'S DATE OF BIRTH MM DD YY SEX M F

b. OTHER INSURED'S DATE OF BIRTH MM DD YY SEX M F

b. AUTO ACCIDENT? YES NO PLACE (State)

b. EMPLOYER'S NAME OR SCHOOL NAME

c. EMPLOYER'S NAME OR SCHOOL NAME

c. OTHER ACCIDENT? YES NO

c. INSURANCE PLAN NAME OR PROGRAM NAME

d. INSURANCE PLAN NAME OR PROGRAM NAME

10d. RESERVED FOR LOCAL USE

d. IS THERE ANOTHER HEALTH BENEFIT PLAN? YES NO *If yes*, return to and complete item 9 a-d.

READ BACK OF FORM BEFORE COMPLETING & SIGNING THIS FORM.

12. PATIENT'S OR AUTHORIZED PERSON'S SIGNATURE I authorize the release of any medical or other information necessary to process this claim. I also request payment of government benefits either to myself or to the party who accepts assignment below.

SIGNED ______ DATE ______

13. INSURED'S OR AUTHORIZED PERSON'S SIGNATURE I authorize payment of medical benefits to the undersigned physician or supplier for services described below.

SIGNED ______

14. DATE OF CURRENT: MM DD YY ILLNESS (First symptom) OR INJURY (Accident) OR PREGNANCY(LMP)

15. IF PATIENT HAS HAD SAME OR SIMILAR ILLNESS. GIVE FIRST DATE MM DD YY

16. DATES PATIENT UNABLE TO WORK IN CURRENT OCCUPATION FROM MM DD YY TO MM DD YY

17. NAME OF REFERRING PHYSICIAN OR OTHER SOURCE

17a. I.D. NUMBER OF REFERRING PHYSICIAN

18. HOSPITALIZATION DATES RELATED TO CURRENT SERVICES FROM MM DD YY TO MM DD YY

19. RESERVED FOR LOCAL USE

20. OUTSIDE LAB? YES NO $ CHARGES

21. DIAGNOSIS OR NATURE OF ILLNESS OR INJURY. (RELATE ITEMS 1,2,3 OR 4 TO ITEM 24E BY LINE)

1. ____ . __

2. ____ . __

3. ____ . __

4. ____ . __

22. MEDICAID RESUBMISSION CODE ORIGINAL REF. NO.

23. PRIOR AUTHORIZATION NUMBER

24. A DATE(S) OF SERVICE From MM DD YY	To MM DD YY	B Place of Service	C Type of Service	D PROCEDURES, SERVICES, OR SUPPLIES (Explain Unusual Circumstances) CPT/HCPCS | MODIFIER	E DIAGNOSIS CODE	F $ CHARGES	G DAYS OR UNITS	H EPSDT Family Plan	I EMG	J COB	K RESERVED FOR LOCAL USE
1											
2											
3											
4											
5											
6											

25. FEDERAL TAX I.D. NUMBER SSN EIN

26. PATIENT'S ACCOUNT NO.

27. ACCEPT ASSIGNMENT? (For govt. claims, see back) YES NO

28. TOTAL CHARGE $

29. AMOUNT PAID $

30. BALANCE DUE $

31. SIGNATURE OF PHYSICIAN OR SUPPLIER INCLUDING DEGREES OR CREDENTIALS (I certify that the statements on the reverse apply to this bill and are made a part thereof.)

SIGNED DATE

32. NAME AND ADDRESS OF FACILITY WHERE SERVICES WERE RENDERED (If other than home or office)

33. PHYSICIAN'S, SUPPLIER'S BILLING NAME, ADDRESS, ZIP CODE & PHONE #

PIN# GRP#

(APPROVED BY AMA COUNCIL ON MEDICAL SERVICE 8/88)

PLEASE PRINT OR TYPE

FORM HCFA-1500 (12-90), FORM RRB-1500, FORM OWCP-1500

PLEASE DO NOT STAPLE IN THIS AREA

APPROVED OMB-0938-0008

PICA

HEALTH INSURANCE CLAIM FORM

PICA

1. MEDICARE (Medicare #) MEDICAID (Medicaid #) CHAMPUS (Sponsor's SSN) CHAMPVA (VA File #) GROUP HEALTH PLAN (SSN or ID) FECA BLK LUNG (SSN) OTHER (ID)

1a. INSURED'S I.D. NUMBER (FOR PROGRAM IN ITEM 1)

2. PATIENT'S NAME (Last Name, First Name, Middle Initial)

3. PATIENT'S BIRTH DATE MM DD YY SEX M F

4. INSURED'S NAME (Last Name, First Name, Middle Initial)

5. PATIENT'S ADDRESS (No., Street)

6. PATIENT RELATIONSHIP TO INSURED Self Spouse Child Other

7. INSURED'S ADDRESS (No., Street)

CITY STATE

8. PATIENT STATUS Single Married Other

Employed Full-Time Student Part-Time Student

CITY STATE

ZIP CODE TELEPHONE (Include Area Code) ( )

ZIP CODE TELEPHONE (INCLUDE AREA CODE) ( )

9. OTHER INSURED'S NAME (Last Name, First Name, Middle Initial)

10. IS PATIENT'S CONDITION RELATED TO:

11. INSURED'S POLICY GROUP OR FECA NUMBER

a. OTHER INSURED'S POLICY OR GROUP NUMBER

a. EMPLOYMENT? (CURRENT OR PREVIOUS) YES NO

a. INSURED'S DATE OF BIRTH MM DD YY SEX M F

b. OTHER INSURED'S DATE OF BIRTH MM DD YY SEX M F

b. AUTO ACCIDENT? YES NO PLACE (State)

b. EMPLOYER'S NAME OR SCHOOL NAME

c. EMPLOYER'S NAME OR SCHOOL NAME

c. OTHER ACCIDENT? YES NO

c. INSURANCE PLAN NAME OR PROGRAM NAME

d. INSURANCE PLAN NAME OR PROGRAM NAME

10d. RESERVED FOR LOCAL USE

d. IS THERE ANOTHER HEALTH BENEFIT PLAN? YES NO *If yes*, return to and complete item 9 a-d.

READ BACK OF FORM BEFORE COMPLETING & SIGNING THIS FORM.

12. PATIENT'S OR AUTHORIZED PERSON'S SIGNATURE I authorize the release of any medical or other information necessary to process this claim. I also request payment of government benefits either to myself or to the party who accepts assignment below.

SIGNED ______ DATE ______

13. INSURED'S OR AUTHORIZED PERSON'S SIGNATURE I authorize payment of medical benefits to the undersigned physician or supplier for services described below.

SIGNED ______

14. DATE OF CURRENT: MM DD YY ILLNESS (First symptom) OR INJURY (Accident) OR PREGNANCY(LMP)

15. IF PATIENT HAS HAD SAME OR SIMILAR ILLNESS. GIVE FIRST DATE MM DD YY

16. DATES PATIENT UNABLE TO WORK IN CURRENT OCCUPATION FROM MM DD YY TO MM DD YY

17. NAME OF REFERRING PHYSICIAN OR OTHER SOURCE

17a. I.D. NUMBER OF REFERRING PHYSICIAN

18. HOSPITALIZATION DATES RELATED TO CURRENT SERVICES FROM MM DD YY TO MM DD YY

19. RESERVED FOR LOCAL USE

20. OUTSIDE LAB? YES NO $ CHARGES

21. DIAGNOSIS OR NATURE OF ILLNESS OR INJURY. (RELATE ITEMS 1,2,3 OR 4 TO ITEM 24E BY LINE)

1. ____ . __

2. ____ . __

3. ____ . __

4. ____ . __

22. MEDICAID RESUBMISSION CODE ORIGINAL REF. NO.

23. PRIOR AUTHORIZATION NUMBER

24. A DATE(S) OF SERVICE From MM DD YY To MM DD YY	B Place of Service	C Type of Service	D PROCEDURES, SERVICES, OR SUPPLIES (Explain Unusual Circumstances) CPT/HCPCS MODIFIER	E DIAGNOSIS CODE	F $ CHARGES	G DAYS OR UNITS	H EPSDT Family Plan	I EMG	J COB	K RESERVED FOR LOCAL USE
1										
2										
3										
4										
5										
6										

25. FEDERAL TAX I.D. NUMBER SSN EIN

26. PATIENT'S ACCOUNT NO.

27. ACCEPT ASSIGNMENT? (For govt. claims, see back) YES NO

28. TOTAL CHARGE $

29. AMOUNT PAID $

30. BALANCE DUE $

31. SIGNATURE OF PHYSICIAN OR SUPPLIER INCLUDING DEGREES OR CREDENTIALS (I certify that the statements on the reverse apply to this bill and are made a part thereof.)

SIGNED DATE

32. NAME AND ADDRESS OF FACILITY WHERE SERVICES WERE RENDERED (If other than home or office)

33. PHYSICIAN'S, SUPPLIER'S BILLING NAME, ADDRESS, ZIP CODE & PHONE #

PIN# GRP#

(APPROVED BY AMA COUNCIL ON MEDICAL SERVICE 8/88)

PLEASE PRINT OR TYPE

FORM HCFA-1500 (12-90), FORM RRB-1500, FORM OWCP-1500

DOCFORM

	OFFICE/OUTPATIENT		CONSULTATION	
	New(3)	Established(2)	Office/O.P.(3)	Confirm(3)
Minimal Service		99211		
HISTORY				
Problem Focused	99201	99212	99241	99271
Exp/Prob Focused	99202	99213	99242	99272
Detailed	99203	99214	99243	99273
Comprehensive	99204/5	99215	99244/5	99274/5
EXAMINATION				
Problem Focused	99201	99212	99241	99271
Exp/Prob Focused	99202	99213	99242	99272
Detailed	99203	99214	99243	99273
Comprehensive	99204/5	99215	99244/5	99274/5
MEDICAL DECISION MAKING				
Straight Forward	99201/2	99212	99241/2	99271/2
Low Complexity	99203	99213	99243	99273
Mod Complexity	99204	99214	99244	99274
High Complexity	99205	99215	99245	99275

TIME: Total ________ **Counsel/Coord. of Care:** ________

10 minutes	99201	99212		
15		99213	99241	
20	99202			
25		99214		
30	99203		99242	
40		99215	99243	
45	99204			
60	99205		99244	
80			99245	

Patient Name: ________________________

Date: ________ **Physician's signature:** ________________

DOCFORM

	CONSULTATION			EMERG	INPATIENT	
	In-Pat(3)	F/Up(2)	Confirm(3)	New/Est(3)	Initial(3)	Sub(2)
HISTORY						
Problem Focused	99251	99261	99271	99281		99231
Exp/Prob Focused	99252	99262	99272	99282/3		99232
Detailed	99253	99263	99273	99284		99233
Comprehensive	99254/5		99274/5	99285	99221/2/3	
EXAMINATION						
Problem	99251	99261	99271	99281		99231
Exp/Prob Focused	99252	99262	99272	99282/3		99232
Detailed	99253	99263	99273	99284		99233
Comprehensive	99254/5		99274/5	99285	99221/2/3	
MEDICAL DECISION MAKING						
Straight Forward	99251/2	99261	99271/2	99281		99231
Low Complexity	99253	99261	99273	99282	99221	99231
Low/Mod Comp				99283		
Mod Complexity	99254	99262	99274	99284	99222	99232
High Complexity	99255	99263	99275	99285	99223	99233

TIME: Total ________ **Counsel/Coord. of Care** ________

	In-Pat(3)	F/Up(2)	Confirm(3)	New/Est(3)	Initial(3)	Sub(2)
10 minutes		99261				99231
15						
20	99251	99262				
25						99232
30		99263				
35						99233
40	99252					
55	99253					
80	99254					
110	99255					

Patient Name: ____________________

Date: ____________ **Physician's signature:** ____________________

DOCFORM

	OFFICE/OUTPATIENT		CONSULTATION	
	New(3)	Established(2)	Office/O.P.(3)	Confirm(3)
Minimal Service		99211		
HISTORY				
Problem Focused	99201	99212	99241	99271
Exp/Prob Focused	99202	99213	99242	99272
Detailed	99203	99214	99243	99273
Comprehensive	99204/5	99215	99244/5	99274/5
EXAMINATION				
Problem Focused	99201	99212	99241	99271
Exp/Prob Focused	99202	99213	99242	99272
Detailed	99203	99214	99243	99273
Comprehensive	99204/5	99215	99244/5	99274/5
MEDICAL DECISION MAKING				
Straight Forward	99201/2	99212	99241/2	99271/2
Low Complexity	99203	99213	99243	99273
Mod Complexity	99204	99214	99244	99274
High Complexity	99205	99215	99245	99275
TIME: Total ________	**Counsel/Coord. of Care:** ________			
10 minutes	99201	99212		
15		99213	99241	
20	99202			
25		99214		
30	99203		99242	
40		99215	99243	
45	99204			
60	99205		99244	
80			99245	

Patient Name: ____________________

Date: ____________ **Physician's signature:** ____________________

DOCFORM

	CONSULTATION			EMERG	INPATIENT	
	In-Pat(3)	F/Up(2)	Confirm(3)	New/Est(3)	Initial(3)	Sub(2)

HISTORY

	In-Pat(3)	F/Up(2)	Confirm(3)	New/Est(3)	Initial(3)	Sub(2)
Problem Focused	99251	99261	99271	99281		99231
Exp/Prob Focused	99252	99262	99272	99282/3		99232
Detailed	99253	99263	99273	99284		99233
Comprehensive	99254/5		99274/5	99285	99221/2/3	

EXAMINATION

	In-Pat(3)	F/Up(2)	Confirm(3)	New/Est(3)	Initial(3)	Sub(2)
Problem	99251	99261	99271	99281		99231
Exp/Prob Focused	99252	99262	99272	99282/3		99232
Detailed	99253	99263	99273	99284		99233
Comprehensive	99254/5		99274/5	99285	99221/2/3	

MEDICAL DECISION MAKING

	In-Pat(3)	F/Up(2)	Confirm(3)	New/Est(3)	Initial(3)	Sub(2)
Straight Forward	99251/2	99261	99271/2	99281		99231
Low Complexity	99253	99261	99273	99282	99221	99231
Low/Mod Comp				99283		
Mod Complexity	99254	99262	99274	99284	99222	99232
High Complexity	99255	99263	99275	99285	99223	99233

TIME: Total ________ **Counsel/Coord. of Care** ________

	In-Pat(3)	F/Up(2)	Confirm(3)	New/Est(3)	Initial(3)	Sub(2)
10 minutes		99261				99231
15						
20	99251	99262				
25						99232
30		99263				
35						99233
40	99252					
55	99253					
80	99254					
110	99255					

Patient Name: ____________________

Date: ____________ **Physician's signature:** ____________________

©MedBooks P.O. Box 670308 Houston, Texas 77267-0308 1-800-443-7397

DOCFORM

	OFFICE/OUTPATIENT		CONSULTATION	
	New(3)	Established(2)	Office/O.P.(3)	Confirm(3)
Minimal Service		99211		
HISTORY				
Problem Focused	99201	99212	99241	99271
Exp/Prob Focused	99202	99213	99242	99272
Detailed	99203	99214	99243	99273
Comprehensive	99204/5	99215	99244/5	99274/5
EXAMINATION				
Problem Focused	99201	99212	99241	99271
Exp/Prob Focused	99202	99213	99242	99272
Detailed	99203	99214	99243	99273
Comprehensive	99204/5	99215	99244/5	99274/5
MEDICAL DECISION MAKING				
Straight Forward	99201/2	99212	99241/2	99271/2
Low Complexity	99203	99213	99243	99273
Mod Complexity	99204	99214	99244	99274
High Complexity	99205	99215	99245	99275

TIME: Total ______ **Counsel/Coord. of Care:** ______

10 minutes	99201	99212		
15		99213	99241	
20	99202			
25		99214		
30	99203		99242	
40		99215	99243	
45	99204			
60	99205		99244	
80			99245	

Patient Name: ______

Date: ______ **Physician's signature:** ______

DOCFORM

	CONSULTATION			EMERG	INPATIENT	
	In-Pat(3)	F/Up(2)	Confirm(3)	New/Est(3)	Initial(3)	Sub(2)
HISTORY						
Problem Focused	99251	99261	99271	99281		99231
Exp/Prob Focused	99252	99262	99272	99282/3		99232
Detailed	99253	99263	99273	99284		99233
Comprehensive	99254/5		99274/5	99285	99221/2/3	
EXAMINATION						
Problem	99251	99261	99271	99281		99231
Exp/Prob Focused	99252	99262	99272	99282/3		99232
Detailed	99253	99263	99273	99284		99233
Comprehensive	99254/5		99274/5	99285	99221/2/3	
MEDICAL DECISION MAKING						
Straight Forward	99251/2	99261	99271/2	99281		99231
Low Complexity	99253	99261	99273	99282	99221	99231
Low/Mod Comp				99283		
Mod Complexity	99254	99262	99274	99284	99222	99232
High Complexity	99255	99263	99275	99285	99223	99233

TIME: Total ____________ **Counsel/Coord. of Care** ____________

	In-Pat(3)	F/Up(2)	Confirm(3)	New/Est(3)	Initial(3)	Sub(2)
10 minutes		99261				99231
15						
20	99251	99262				
25						99232
30		99263				
35						99233
40	99252					
55	99253					
80	99254					
110	99255					

Patient Name: ______________________________

Date: ____________ **Physician's signature:** ____________________

©MedBooks P.O. Box 670308 Houston, Texas 77267-0308 1-800-443-7397

DOCFORM

	OFFICE/OUTPATIENT		CONSULTATION	
	New(3)	Established(2)	Office/O.P.(3)	Confirm(3)
Minimal Service		99211		
HISTORY				
Problem Focused	99201	99212	99241	99271
Exp/Prob Focused	99202	99213	99242	99272
Detailed	99203	99214	99243	99273
Comprehensive	99204/5	99215	99244/5	99274/5
EXAMINATION				
Problem Focused	99201	99212	99241	99271
Exp/Prob Focused	99202	99213	99242	99272
Detailed	99203	99214	99243	99273
Comprehensive	99204/5	99215	99244/5	99274/5
MEDICAL DECISION MAKING				
Straight Forward	99201/2	99212	99241/2	99271/2
Low Complexity	99203	99213	99243	99273
Mod Complexity	99204	99214	99244	99274
High Complexity	99205	99215	99245	99275
TIME: Total ________		Counsel/Coord. of Care: ________		
10 minutes	99201	99212		
15		99213	99241	
20	99202			
25		99214		
30	99203		99242	
40		99215	99243	
45	99204			
60	99205		99244	
80			99245	

Patient Name: ______________________________

Date: ______________ **Physician's signature:** ______________________

DOCFORM

	CONSULTATION			EMERG	INPATIENT	
	In-Pat(3)	F/Up(2)	Confirm(3)	New/Est(3)	Initial(3)	Sub(2)
HISTORY						
Problem Focused	99251	99261	99271	99281		99231
Exp/Prob Focused	99252	99262	99272	99282/3		99232
Detailed	99253	99263	99273	99284		99233
Comprehensive	99254/5		99274/5	99285	99221/2/3	
EXAMINATION						
Problem	99251	99261	99271	99281		99231
Exp/Prob Focused	99252	99262	99272	99282/3		99232
Detailed	99253	99263	99273	99284		99233
Comprehensive	99254/5		99274/5	99285	99221/2/3	
MEDICAL DECISION MAKING						
Straight Forward	99251/2	99261	99271/2	99281		99231
Low Complexity	99253	99261	99273	99282	99221	99231
Low/Mod Comp				99283		
Mod Complexity	99254	99262	99274	99284	99222	99232
High Complexity	99255	99263	99275	99285	99223	99233

TIME: Total ______________ **Counsel/Coord. of Care** ______________

	In-Pat(3)	F/Up(2)	Confirm(3)	New/Est(3)	Initial(3)	Sub(2)
10 minutes		99261				99231
15						
20	99251	99262				
25						99232
30		99263				
35						99233
40	99252					
55	99253					
80	99254					
110	99255					

Patient Name: ______________________________

Date: ______________ **Physician's signature:** ______________________

©MedBooks P.O. Box 670308 Houston, Texas 77267-0308 1-800-443-7397

DOCFORM

	OFFICE/OUTPATIENT		CONSULTATION	
	New(3)	Established(2)	Office/O.P.(3)	Confirm(3)
Minimal Service		99211		
HISTORY				
Problem Focused	99201	99212	99241	99271
Exp/Prob Focused	99202	99213	99242	99272
Detailed	99203	99214	99243	99273
Comprehensive	99204/5	99215	99244/5	99274/5
EXAMINATION				
Problem Focused	99201	99212	99241	99271
Exp/Prob Focused	99202	99213	99242	99272
Detailed	99203	99214	99243	99273
Comprehensive	99204/5	99215	99244/5	99274/5
MEDICAL DECISION MAKING				
Straight Forward	99201/2	99212	99241/2	99271/2
Low Complexity	99203	99213	99243	99273
Mod Complexity	99204	99214	99244	99274
High Complexity	99205	99215	99245	99275
TIME: Total ________		**Counsel/Coord. of Care:** ________		
10 minutes	99201	99212		
15		99213	99241	
20	99202			
25		99214		
30	99203		99242	
40		99215	99243	
45	99204			
60	99205		99244	
80			99245	

Patient Name: ________________________________

Date: ____________ **Physician's signature:** ____________________

DOCFORM

	CONSULTATION			EMERG	INPATIENT	
	In-Pat(3)	F/Up(2)	Confirm(3)	New/Est(3)	Initial(3)	Sub(2)
HISTORY						
Problem Focused	99251	99261	99271	99281		99231
Exp/Prob Focused	99252	99262	99272	99282/3		99232
Detailed	99253	99263	99273	99284		99233
Comprehensive	99254/5		99274/5	99285	99221/2/3	
EXAMINATION						
Problem	99251	99261	99271	99281		99231
Exp/Prob Focused	99252	99262	99272	99282/3		99232
Detailed	99253	99263	99273	99284		99233
Comprehensive	99254/5		99274/5	99285	99221/2/3	
MEDICAL DECISION MAKING						
Straight Forward	99251/2	99261	99271/2	99281		99231
Low Complexity	99253	99261	99273	99282	99221	99231
Low/Mod Comp				99283		
Mod Complexity	99254	99262	99274	99284	99222	99232
High Complexity	99255	99263	99275	99285	99223	99233

TIME: Total ____________ **Counsel/Coord. of Care** ____________

10 minutes		99261				99231
15						
20	99251	99262				
25						99232
30		99263				
35						99233
40	99252					
55	99253					
80	99254					
110	99255					

Patient Name: ______________________________

Date: ____________ **Physician's signature:** ____________

DOCFORM

	OFFICE/OUTPATIENT		CONSULTATION	
	New(3)	Established(2)	Office/O.P.(3)	Confirm(3)
Minimal Service		99211		
HISTORY				
Problem Focused	99201	99212	99241	99271
Exp/Prob Focused	99202	99213	99242	99272
Detailed	99203	99214	99243	99273
Comprehensive	99204/5	99215	99244/5	99274/5
EXAMINATION				
Problem Focused	99201	99212	99241	99271
Exp/Prob Focused	99202	99213	99242	99272
Detailed	99203	99214	99243	99273
Comprehensive	99204/5	99215	99244/5	99274/5
MEDICAL DECISION MAKING				
Straight Forward	99201/2	99212	99241/2	99271/2
Low Complexity	99203	99213	99243	99273
Mod Complexity	99204	99214	99244	99274
High Complexity	99205	99215	99245	99275

TIME: Total ________ **Counsel/Coord. of Care:** ________

10 minutes	99201	99212		
15		99213	99241	
20	99202			
25		99214		
30	99203		99242	
40		99215	99243	
45	99204			
60	99205		99244	
80			99245	

Patient Name: ____________________

Date: ____________ **Physician's signature:** ____________

DOCFORM

	CONSULTATION			EMERG	INPATIENT	
	In-Pat(3)	F/Up(2)	Confirm(3)	New/Est(3)	Initial(3)	Sub(2)
HISTORY						
Problem Focused	99251	99261	99271	99281		99231
Exp/Prob Focused	99252	99262	99272	99282/3		99232
Detailed	99253	99263	99273	99284		99233
Comprehensive	99254/5		99274/5	99285	99221/2/3	
EXAMINATION						
Problem	99251	99261	99271	99281		99231
Exp/Prob Focused	99252	99262	99272	99282/3		99232
Detailed	99253	99263	99273	99284		99233
Comprehensive	99254/5		99274/5	99285	99221/2/3	
MEDICAL DECISION MAKING						
Straight Forward	99251/2	99261	99271/2	99281		99231
Low Complexity	99253	99261	99273	99282	99221	99231
Low/Mod Comp				99283		
Mod Complexity	99254	99262	99274	99284	99222	99232
High Complexity	99255	99263	99275	99285	99223	99233

TIME: Total ______ **Counsel/Coord. of Care** ______

	In-Pat(3)	F/Up(2)	Confirm(3)	New/Est(3)	Initial(3)	Sub(2)
10 minutes		99261				99231
15						
20	99251	99262				
25						99232
30		99263				
35						99233
40	99252					
55	99253					
80	99254					
110	99255					

Patient Name: ______________________________

Date: ______________ **Physician's signature:** ______________________

DOCFORM

	OFFICE/OUTPATIENT		CONSULTATION	
	New(3)	Established(2)	Office/O.P.(3)	Confirm(3)
Minimal Service		99211		
HISTORY				
Problem Focused	99201	99212	99241	99271
Exp/Prob Focused	99202	99213	99242	99272
Detailed	99203	99214	99243	99273
Comprehensive	99204/5	99215	99244/5	99274/5
EXAMINATION				
Problem Focused	99201	99212	99241	99271
Exp/Prob Focused	99202	99213	99242	99272
Detailed	99203	99214	99243	99273
Comprehensive	99204/5	99215	99244/5	99274/5
MEDICAL DECISION MAKING				
Straight Forward	99201/2	99212	99241/2	99271/2
Low Complexity	99203	99213	99243	99273
Mod Complexity	99204	99214	99244	99274
High Complexity	99205	99215	99245	99275

TIME: Total __________ **Counsel/Coord. of Care:** __________

10 minutes	99201	99212		
15		99213	99241	
20	99202			
25		99214		
30	99203		99242	
40		99215	99243	
45	99204			
60	99205		99244	
80			99245	

Patient Name: ____________________

Date: __________ **Physician's signature:** __________

DOCFORM

	CONSULTATION			EMERG	INPATIENT	
	In-Pat(3)	F/Up(2)	Confirm(3)	New/Est(3)	Initial(3)	Sub(2)
HISTORY						
Problem Focused	99251	99261	99271	99281		99231
Exp/Prob Focused	99252	99262	99272	99282/3		99232
Detailed	99253	99263	99273	99284		99233
Comprehensive	99254/5		99274/5	99285	99221/2/3	
EXAMINATION						
Problem	99251	99261	99271	99281		99231
Exp/Prob Focused	99252	99262	99272	99282/3		99232
Detailed	99253	99263	99273	99284		99233
Comprehensive	99254/5		99274/5	99285	99221/2/3	
MEDICAL DECISION MAKING						
Straight Forward	99251/2	99261	99271/2	99281		99231
Low Complexity	99253	99261	99273	99282	99221	99231
Low/Mod Comp				99283		
Mod Complexity	99254	99262	99274	99284	99222	99232
High Complexity	99255	99263	99275	99285	99223	99233

TIME: Total __________ **Counsel/Coord. of Care** __________

	In-Pat(3)	F/Up(2)	Confirm(3)	New/Est(3)	Initial(3)	Sub(2)
10 minutes		99261				99231
15						
20	99251	99262				
25						99232
30		99263				
35						99233
40	99252					
55	99253					
80	99254					
110	99255					

Patient Name: ____________________

Date: __________ **Physician's signature:** ____________________

©MedBooks P.O. Box 670308 Houston, Texas 77267-0308 1-800-443-7397

DOCFORM

	OFFICE/OUTPATIENT		CONSULTATION	
	New(3)	Established(2)	Office/O.P.(3)	Confirm(3)
Minimal Service		99211		
HISTORY				
Problem Focused	99201	99212	99241	99271
Exp/Prob Focused	99202	99213	99242	99272
Detailed	99203	99214	99243	99273
Comprehensive	99204/5	99215	99244/5	99274/5
EXAMINATION				
Problem Focused	99201	99212	99241	99271
Exp/Prob Focused	99202	99213	99242	99272
Detailed	99203	99214	99243	99273
Comprehensive	99204/5	99215	99244/5	99274/5
MEDICAL DECISION MAKING				
Straight Forward	99201/2	99212	99241/2	99271/2
Low Complexity	99203	99213	99243	99273
Mod Complexity	99204	99214	99244	99274
High Complexity	99205	99215	99245	99275
TIME: Total ______		**Counsel/Coord. of Care:** ______		
10 minutes	99201	99212		
15		99213	99241	
20	99202			
25		99214		
30	99203		99242	
40		99215	99243	
45	99204			
60	99205		99244	
80			99245	

Patient Name: ______________________________

Date: ______________ **Physician's signature:** ______________________

DOCFORM

	CONSULTATION			EMERG	INPATIENT	
	In-Pat(3)	F/Up(2)	Confirm(3)	New/Est(3)	Initial(3)	Sub(2)
HISTORY						
Problem Focused	99251	99261	99271	99281		99231
Exp/Prob Focused	99252	99262	99272	99282/3		99232
Detailed	99253	99263	99273	99284		99233
Comprehensive	99254/5		99274/5	99285	99221/2/3	
EXAMINATION						
Problem	99251	99261	99271	99281		99231
Exp/Prob Focused	99252	99262	99272	99282/3		99232
Detailed	99253	99263	99273	99284		99233
Comprehensive	99254/5		99274/5	99285	99221/2/3	
MEDICAL DECISION MAKING						
Straight Forward	99251/2	99261	99271/2	99281		99231
Low Complexity	99253	99261	99273	99282	99221	99231
Low/Mod Comp				99283		
Mod Complexity	99254	99262	99274	99284	99222	99232
High Complexity	99255	99263	99275	99285	99223	99233

TIME: Total __________ **Counsel/Coord. of Care** __________

	In-Pat(3)	F/Up(2)	Confirm(3)	New/Est(3)	Initial(3)	Sub(2)
10 minutes		99261				99231
15						
20	99251	99262				
25						99232
30		99263				
35						99233
40	99252					
55	99253					
80	99254					
110	99255					

Patient Name: ____________________

Date: __________ **Physician's signature:** ________________

DOCFORM

	OFFICE/OUTPATIENT		CONSULTATION	
	New(3)	Established(2)	Office/O.P.(3)	Confirm(3)
Minimal Service		99211		
HISTORY				
Problem Focused	99201	99212	99241	99271
Exp/Prob Focused	99202	99213	99242	99272
Detailed	99203	99214	99243	99273
Comprehensive	99204/5	99215	99244/5	99274/5
EXAMINATION				
Problem Focused	99201	99212	99241	99271
Exp/Prob Focused	99202	99213	99242	99272
Detailed	99203	99214	99243	99273
Comprehensive	99204/5	99215	99244/5	99274/5
MEDICAL DECISION MAKING				
Straight Forward	99201/2	99212	99241/2	99271/2
Low Complexity	99203	99213	99243	99273
Mod Complexity	99204	99214	99244	99274
High Complexity	99205	99215	99245	99275

TIME: Total ____________ **Counsel/Coord. of Care:** ____________

10 minutes	99201	99212		
15		99213	99241	
20	99202			
25		99214		
30	99203		99242	
40		99215	99243	
45	99204			
60	99205		99244	
80			99245	

Patient Name: ______________________________

Date: ____________ **Physician's signature:** ______________________

DOCFORM

	CONSULTATION			EMERG	INPATIENT	
	In-Pat(3)	F/Up(2)	Confirm(3)	New/Est(3)	Initial(3)	Sub(2)
HISTORY						
Problem Focused	99251	99261	99271	99281		99231
Exp/Prob Focused	99252	99262	99272	99282/3		99232
Detailed	99253	99263	99273	99284		99233
Comprehensive	99254/5		99274/5	99285	99221/2/3	
EXAMINATION						
Problem	99251	99261	99271	99281		99231
Exp/Prob Focused	99252	99262	99272	99282/3		99232
Detailed	99253	99263	99273	99284		99233
Comprehensive	99254/5		99274/5	99285	99221/2/3	
MEDICAL DECISION MAKING						
Straight Forward	99251/2	99261	99271/2	99281		99231
Low Complexity	99253	99261	99273	99282	99221	99231
Low/Mod Comp				99283		
Mod Complexity	99254	99262	99274	99284	99222	99232
High Complexity	99255	99263	99275	99285	99223	99233

TIME: Total __________ **Counsel/Coord. of Care** __________

	In-Pat(3)	F/Up(2)	Confirm(3)	New/Est(3)	Initial(3)	Sub(2)
10 minutes		99261				99231
15						
20	99251	99262				
25						99232
30		99263				
35						99233
40	99252					
55	99253					
80	99254					
110	99255					

Patient Name: ____________________

Date: __________ **Physician's signature:** ____________________

DOCFORM

	OFFICE/OUTPATIENT		CONSULTATION	
	New(3)	Established(2)	Office/O.P.(3)	Confirm(3)
Minimal Service		99211		
HISTORY				
Problem Focused	99201	99212	99241	99271
Exp/Prob Focused	99202	99213	99242	99272
Detailed	99203	99214	99243	99273
Comprehensive	99204/5	99215	99244/5	99274/5
EXAMINATION				
Problem Focused	99201	99212	99241	99271
Exp/Prob Focused	99202	99213	99242	99272
Detailed	99203	99214	99243	99273
Comprehensive	99204/5	99215	99244/5	99274/5
MEDICAL DECISION MAKING				
Straight Forward	99201/2	99212	99241/2	99271/2
Low Complexity	99203	99213	99243	99273
Mod Complexity	99204	99214	99244	99274
High Complexity	99205	99215	99245	99275

TIME: Total __________ **Counsel/Coord. of Care:** __________

10 minutes	99201	99212		
15		99213	99241	
20	99202			
25		99214		
30	99203		99242	
40		99215	99243	
45	99204			
60	99205		99244	
80			99245	

Patient Name: ____________________

Date: __________ **Physician's signature:** ________________

DOCFORM

	CONSULTATION			EMERG	INPATIENT	
	In-Pat(3)	F/Up(2)	Confirm(3)	New/Est(3)	Initial(3)	Sub(2)
HISTORY						
Problem Focused	99251	99261	99271	99281		99231
Exp/Prob Focused	99252	99262	99272	99282/3		99232
Detailed	99253	99263	99273	99284		99233
Comprehensive	99254/5		99274/5	99285	99221/2/3	
EXAMINATION						
Problem	99251	99261	99271	99281		99231
Exp/Prob Focused	99252	99262	99272	99282/3		99232
Detailed	99253	99263	99273	99284		99233
Comprehensive	99254/5		99274/5	99285	99221/2/3	
MEDICAL DECISION MAKING						
Straight Forward	99251/2	99261	99271/2	99281		99231
Low Complexity	99253	99261	99273	99282	99221	99231
Low/Mod Comp				99283		
Mod Complexity	99254	99262	99274	99284	99222	99232
High Complexity	99255	99263	99275	99285	99223	99233

TIME: Total ____________ Counsel/Coord. of Care ____________

	In-Pat(3)	F/Up(2)	Confirm(3)	New/Est(3)	Initial(3)	Sub(2)
10 minutes		99261				99231
15						
20	99251	99262				
25						99232
30		99263				
35						99233
40	99252					
55	99253					
80	99254					
110	99255					

Patient Name: ____

Date: ______________ **Physician's signature:** ______________________

Do not do these codes @ home.

The following examples are real. They have been given to us by a very generous hospital in Louisiana. We are grateful to them for their time and energy to put these examples together.

Please code the following examples and decide which CPT code you will use, which ICD-9-CM diagnosis code(s) and procedural codes you will use and place these on the forms that follow.

We will go over this in class.
Outpatent coding is a new way of coding, it is ambulatory services.

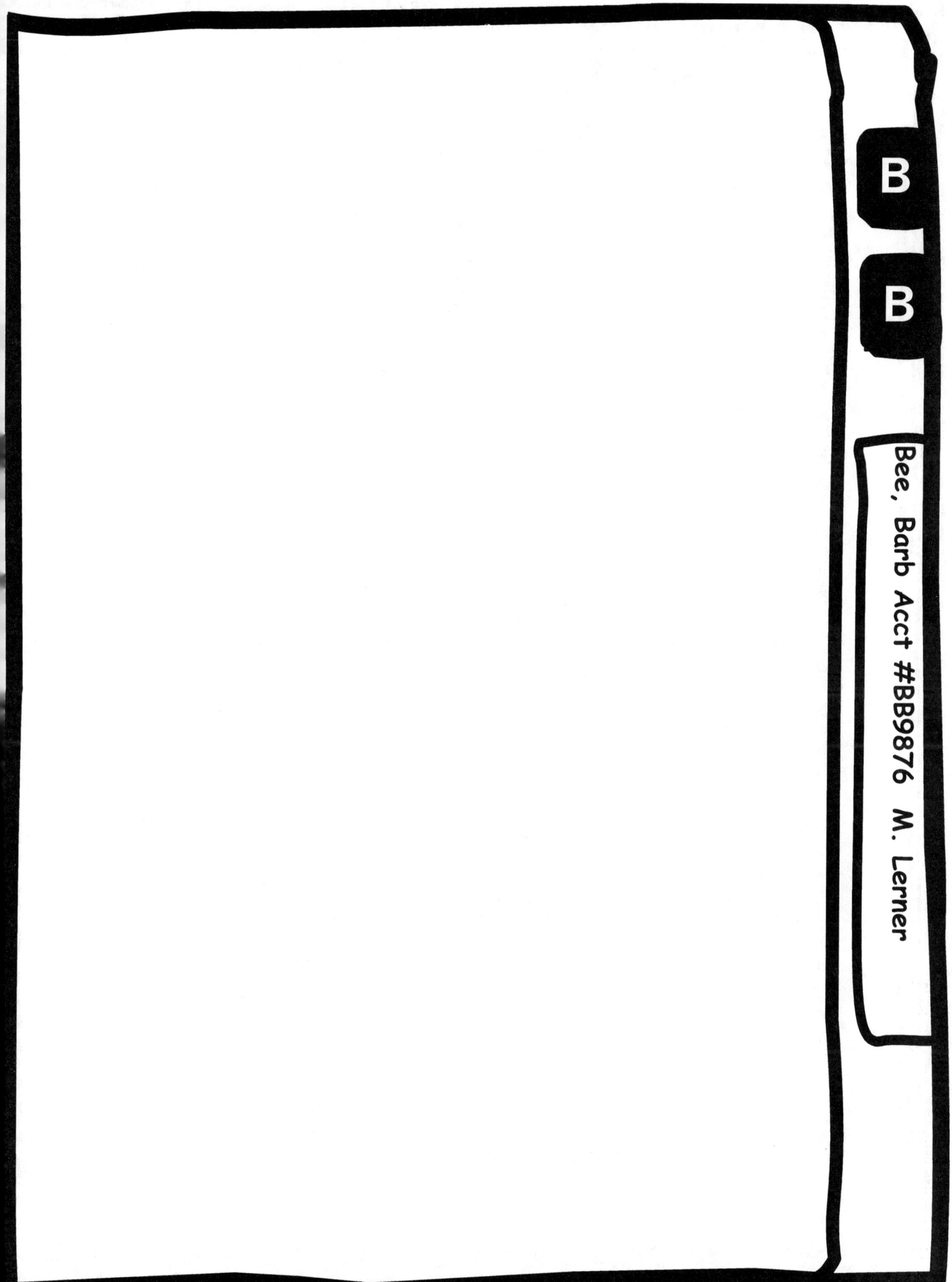
B
B
Bee, Barb Acct #BB9876 M. Lerner

OUTPATIENT RECORD

Account:	Physician:	Phy #:	Registration Date:	Time:	MSV:	Admit Category:	Med Rec. No.
BB9876	M. Lerner	ML871	8/22	07:26		Rad	P55089

PATIENT

Name:				
Barb Bee				
Address: 5618 Logical Street	Religion: presby.	DOB: 09/16	SEX: F	MS:
City: Paynesville	State: TX	Zip: 77777		
Residence Phone: 999-765-0767	County: Broken Toe	Social Security No. 768-09-3758		

EMPLOYER

Name:		
Pampered Chef		
Address: 8756 Cooks Court		
City: Paynesville	State: TX	Zip: 77777
Phone: 999-823-0587	ADM By: sp	Occupation: cook/chef

GUARANTOR

Name:		
Neil Bee		
Address: Same	RELN.	Guarantor No. Y76298
City: Paynesville	State: TX	Zip: 77777
Phone: 999-898-2323	Social Security: 565-09-2415	

EMPLOYER

Name:		
Tenent Insurance		
Address: 8787 Poplar Street		
City: Paynesville	State: TX	Zip: 77777
Phone: 999-876-0123	Occupation: data entry	

INSURANCE

Insurance Company:	Plan #:	Group #:	Policy #:	Policy Holder:	Relation:	Sex:
Tenent Insurance Corporate Office 1180 Security Way Anderton, OK 76987	TI898	YH7654	YH5656	Neil Bee	husband	M

Admit Complaint:	Prvs. Admit This Hospital	Notify In Case Of Emergency:
palpatations	2 weeks ago	Neil Bee

Comments:
last episode lasted 7 hours (see 8/05)

NURSING ASSESMENT

Medications:
verapamil 120 mg none longer used
adenosine

LTT	WT.		T	B/P	P	R
	167		98.7	135/80		

Physician:
M. Lerner

CONSENT TO TREATMENT: I, the undersigned hereby authorize St. Theresa Memorial Hospital to provide such medical care and to administer such laboratory procedures, radiological diagnostic and/or Therapeutic procedures and treatments, including but not limited to administration of pharmaceutical products, infusion or transfusion of blood or blood components, injections and intravenous medication or other therapeutic solutions as in the judgment of the physicians treating the patient may be deemed necessary and advisable. I understand I am entitled to have my own physician treat me, and he (she) will be called upon my request. I understand that a personal physician is to be selected by or on behalf of the patient within 24 hours if hospitalization or further treatment is required, or immediately if complaints arise. RELEASE OF INFORMATION: I hear-by authorize St. Theresa Memorial Hospital to release any information to any organization providing transportation to or from this hospital.

Signed: ______________________ Date: __________ Relationship to Patient ______________

If unable to sign, reason: ______________________________

Witness ______________ Witness ______________ Other Consent ______________

Physician Signature	Page No.	Title:
		Date:

Outpatient Services
St. Theresa's Hospital
Paynesville, Texas 77777

Name: Barb Bee

Case #: P55089

Physician: M. Lerner

Date: 08/22

Anesthetist:

Assistant:

Started:

Ended:

Preoperative Diagnosis: Cardiac Arrhythmia

Postoperative Diagnosis: Same

Operation:

Anesthesia:

INDICATIONS: This 42 year-old female has long standing palpatations. She had a severe episode lasting 7 hours this past weekend. She was already on Verapamil 120 mg. per day. She was found to be in rapid SVT. She was converted with Adenosine.

PROCEDURE: Diagnostic Electrophysiologic Study and Radiofrequency Catheter Ablation

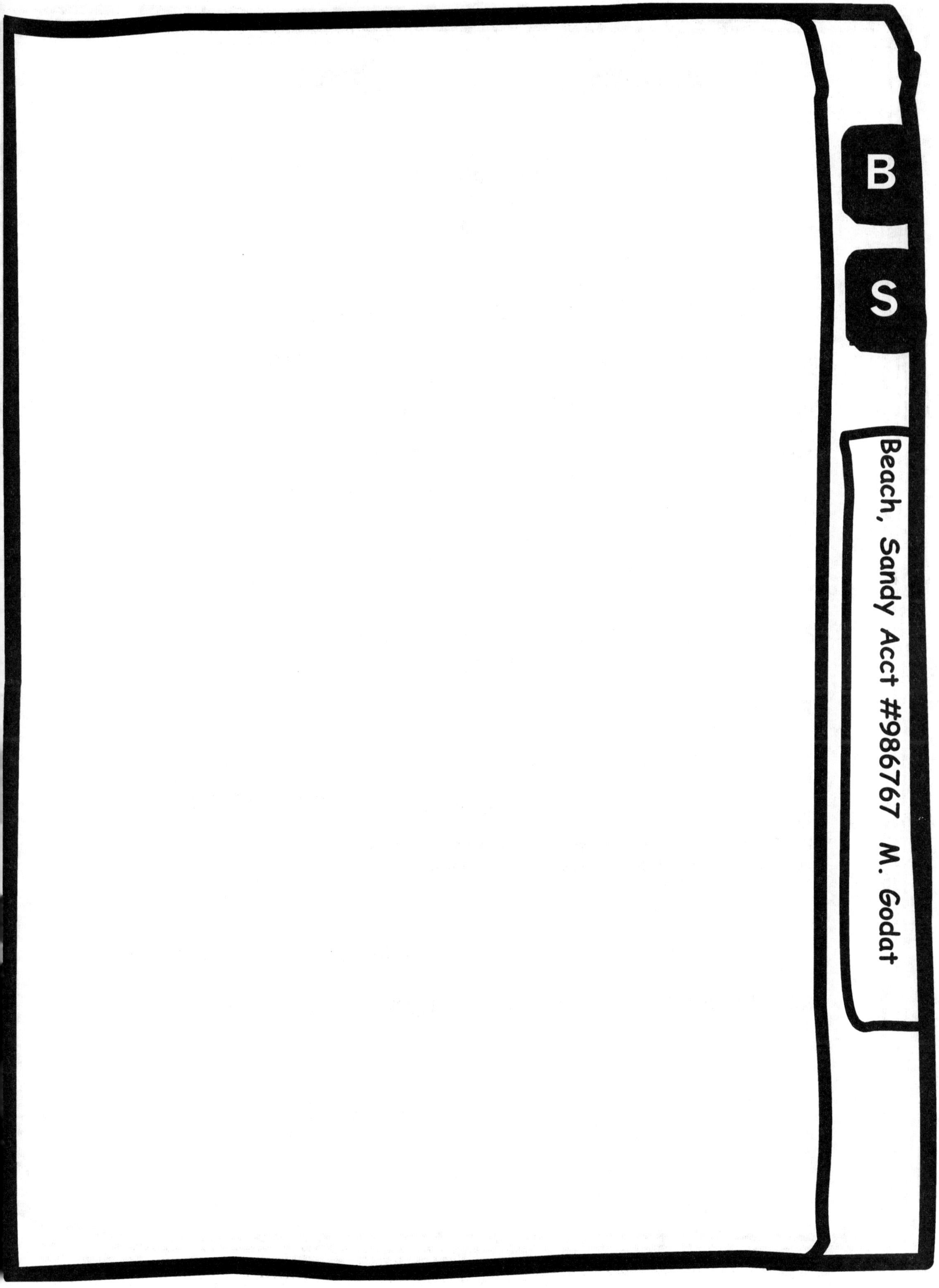
B
S
Beach, Sandy Acct #986767 M. Godat

Outpatient Services
St. Theresa's Hospital
Paynesville, Texas 77777

Name: Sandy Beach **Case #:** P5311J

Physician: M. Godat **Date:** 12/15/

Anesthetist: **Assistant:**

Started: **Ended:**

Preoperative Diagnosis: Equinus deformity of both feet
Cerebral palsy

Postoperative Diagnosis: Equinus deformity of both feet
Cerebral palsy

Operation:

Anesthesia:

INDICATIONS: This 10-year old girl walks on her tip toes. Feet and ankles point down and cannot forcefully be placed at 90 degrees.

PROCEDURE: Bilateral tendon Achilles lengthening.

OUTPATIENT RECORD

Account:	Physician:	Phy #:	Registration Date:	Time:	MSV:	Admit Category:	Med Rec. No.
986767	M. Godat	67654	12/15	10:55			P5311J

PATIENT

Name:				
Sandy Beach				
Address: 67 Tunnel Ave.	Religion: baptist	DOB: 07/06	SEX: F	MS:
City: Paynesville	State: TX	Zip: 77777		
Residence Phone: 999-767-4651	County: Broken Toe	Social Security No. 342-07-9761		

GUARANTOR

Name:		
Pauline and Earl Beach		
Address: Same	RELN. same	Guarantor No. 87J761
City:	State:	Zip:
Phone: same	Social Security: 876-434-1256	

EMPLOYER

Name:		
Address:		
City:	State:	Zip:
Phone:	ADM By: RH	Occupation:
Name: Unysis		
Address: 1111 High Drive		
City: Paynesville	State: TX	Zip: 77777
Phone: 999-767-1782	Occupation: COMPUTER ANALYST	

INSURANCE

Insurance Company:	Plan #:	Group #:	Policy #:	Policy Holder:	Relation:	Sex:
The Best 3407 Corporate Way Anytown, IN 76298	86HT	77HLF	SB1267	Pauline Beach	mother	F

Admit Complaint:	Prvs. Admit This Hospital	Notify In Case Of Emergency:
walks on tip toes	nne	parents see above

Comments:

NURSING ASSESMENT

Medications:
none

LTT	WT.		T	B/P	P	R

Physician:
M. Godat

CONSENT TO TREATMENT: I, the undersigned hereby authorize St. Theresa Memorial Hospital to provide such medical care and to administer such laboratory procedures, radiological diagnostic and/or Therapeutic procedures and treatments, including but not limited to administration of pharmaceutical products, infusion or transfusion of blood or blood components, injections and intravenous medication or other therapeutic solutions as in the judgment of the physicians treating the patient may be deemed necessary and advisable. I understand I am entitled to have my own physician treat me, and he (she) will be called upon my request. I understand that a personal physician is to be selected by or on behalf of the patient within 24 hours if hospitalization or further treatment is required, or immediately if complaints arise. RELEASE OF INFORMATION: I hear-by authorize St. Theresa Memorial Hospital to release any information to any organization providing transportation to or from this hospital.

Signed: ____________________ Date: __________ Relationship to Patient ____________

If unable to sign, reason: ______________________________

Witness ______________ Witness ______________ Other Consent ______________

Physician Signature	Page No.	Title:
		Date:

B

S

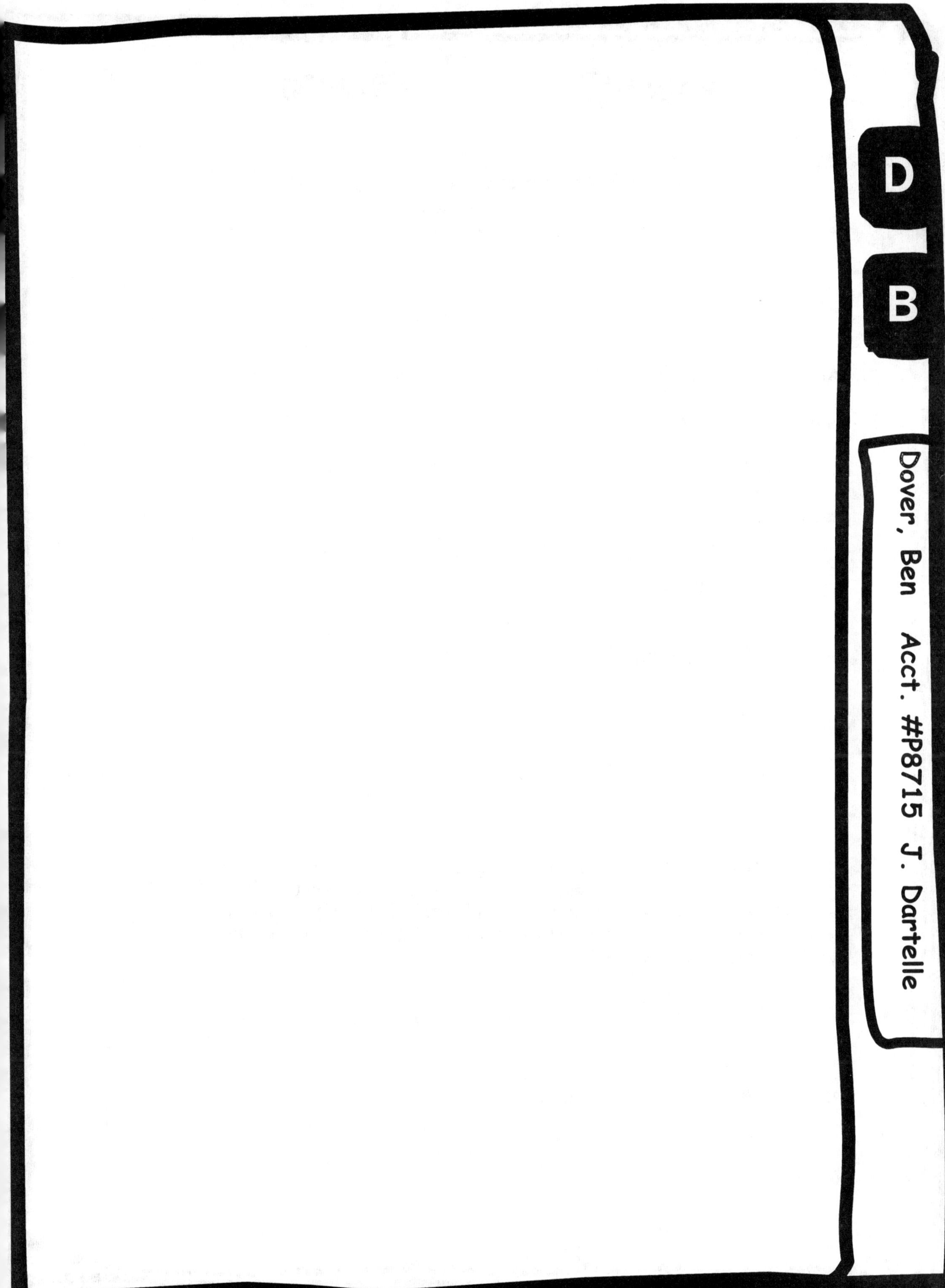
D
B
Dover, Ben Acct. #P8715 J. Dartelle

Outpatient Services
St. Theresa's Hospital
Paynesville, Texas 77777

Name: Ben Dover

Case #: P11334

Physician: B. Dartelle

Date: 2/14/

Anesthetist:

Assistant:

Started:

Ended:

Preoperative Diagnosis: Backache

Postoperative Diagnosis: Spinal Stenosis Lumbar

Operation:

Anesthesia:

INDICATIONS: 74 year old male having pain in both of his legs, right worse than left after walking 2 to 3 hundred feet. This is relieved by 2 to 3 minutes of rest. Patient has Neurogenic Claudication secondary to lumbar spinal Stenosis. Recommend delineation of the magnitude of the problem with Myelography and correction before his symptoms become totally disabling.

PROCEDURE:
1. Contrast Myelogram;
2. C.A.T. Scan

OUTPATIENT RECORD

Account:	Physician:	Phy #:	Registration Date:	Time:	MSV:	Admit Category:	Med Rec. No.
P8715	B. Dartelle	BD8876	2/14	23:00		ER	P11334

PATIENT

Name:				
Ben Dover				
Address: 6525 Haynie Drive	Religion: Cath.	DOB: 07/27	SEX: M	MS:
City: Paynesville	State: TX	Zip: 77777		
Residence Phone: 999-789-0111	County: Broken Toe	Social Security No. 434-27-3197		

GUARANTOR

Name:		
Ben Dover		
Address: Same	RELN.	Guarantor No.
City:	State:	Zip:
Phone:	Social Security:	

EMPLOYER

Name:		
Address:		
City:	State:	Zip:
Phone:	ADM By: sp	Occupation:
Name:		
Address:		
City:	State:	Zip:
Phone:	Occupation:	

INSURANCE

Insurance Company:	Plan #:	Group #:	Policy #:	Policy Holder:	Relation:	Sex:
BCBS Medicare 111 Texas Way Dallas, Texas 76543	MC33	HY66	MC445	Ben Dover	self	M

Admit Complaint:	Prvs. Admit This Hospital	Notify In Case Of Emergency:
pain in legs	none	Rita Hayworth 999-876-8877

Comments:
pain relieved by rest

NURSING ASSESMENT

Medications:
none

LTT	WT.		T	B/P	P	R
	170		98.2	119/76		

Physician:
B. Dartelle

CONSENT TO TREATMENT: I, the undersigned hereby authorize St. Theresa Memorial Hospital to provide such medical care and to administer such laboratory procedures, radiological diagnostic and/or Therapeutic procedures and treatments, including but not limited to administration of pharmaceutical products, infusion or transfusion of blood or blood components, injections and intravenous medication or other therapeutic solutions as in the judgment of the physicians treating the patient may be deemed necessary and advisable. I understand I am entitled to have my own physician treat me, and he (she) will be called upon my request. I understand that a personal physician is to be selected by or on behalf of the patient within 24 hours if hospitalization or further treatment is required, or immediately if complaints arise. RELEASE OF INFORMATION: I hear-by authorize St. Theresa Memorial Hospital to release any information to any organization providing transportation to or from this hospital.

Signed: ______________________ Date: __________ Relationship to Patient ______________

If unable to sign, reason: ______________________________________

Witness ____________________ Witness ____________________ Other Consent ______________

Physician Signature	Page No.	Title:
		Date:

D

B

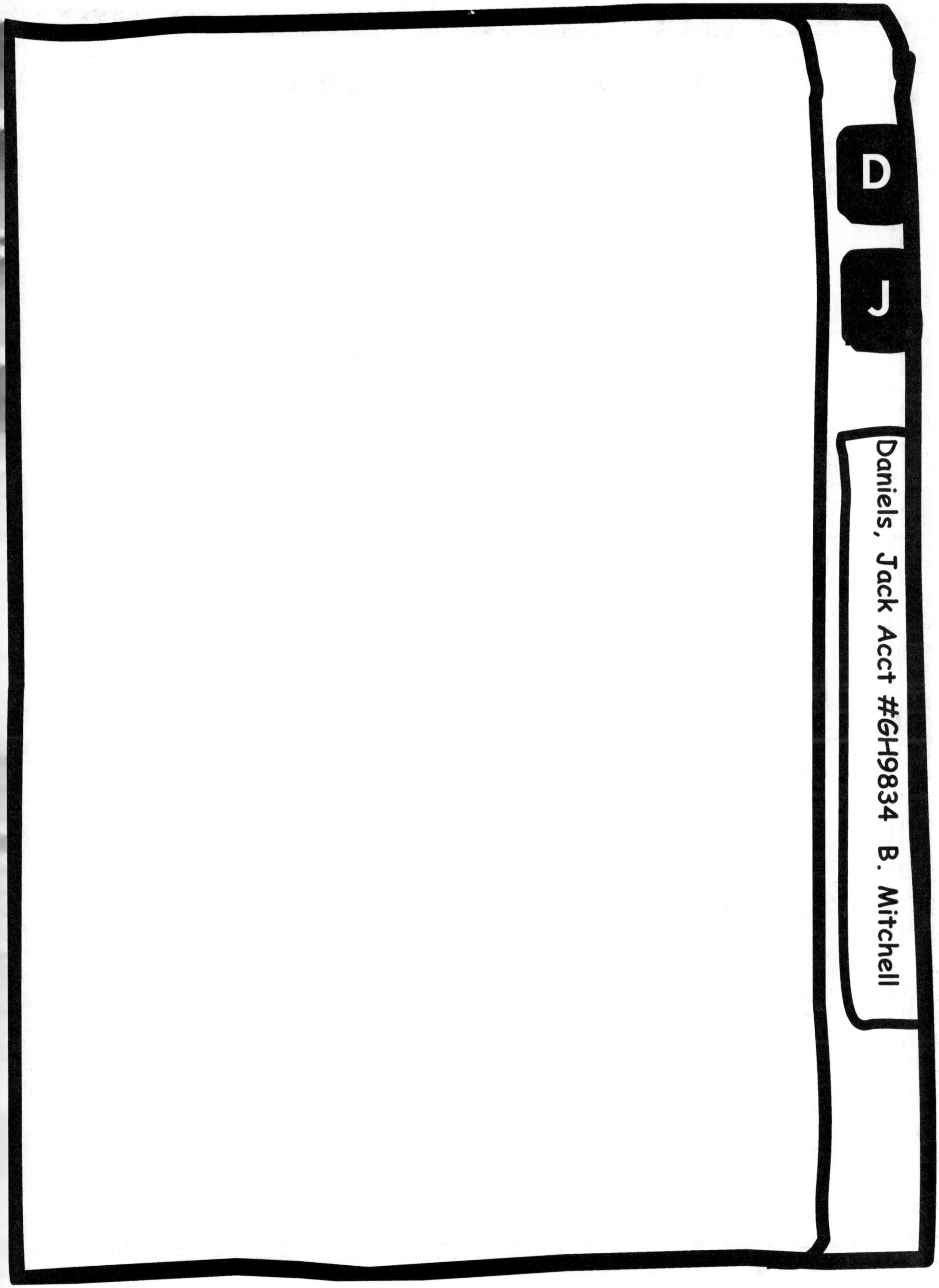
D
J
Daniels, Jack Acct #GH9834 B. Mitchell

Outpatient Services
St. Theresa's Hospital
Paynesville, Texas 77777

Name:	Jack Daniels	**Case #:**	P88112
Physician:	B. Mitchell	**Date:**	8/17/
Anesthetist:		**Assistant:**	
Started:		**Ended:**	

Impressions:

1. Chest Pain of unclear etiology;
2. Moderate increase in creatinine suggesting skeletal muscle injuries;
3. Quadriplegia

Diagnosis:

Operation:

Anesthesia:

INDICATIONS: This 38-year old male presented to the Emergency Room complaining of retrosternal chest tightness. This has been an ongoing process for the last 2 to 3 days. He intermittently gets tightness in his chest associated with very sudden and short-lived SOB. The discomfort in his chest will last 15-20 minutes. He is a quadriplegic although he gets around in a wheelchair on his own and denies any pain, pressure or tightness in his chest, arms, neck or jaws.

PROCEDURE:

OUTPATIENT RECORD

Account:	Physician:	Phy #:	Registration Date:	Time:	MSV:	Admit Category:	Med Rec. No.
GH9834	B. Mitchell	BH876	8/17	12:23		ER	P88112

PATIENT

Name: Jack Daniels

Address:	Religion	DOB:	SEX:	MS:
6520 Hyer Street		8/14	M	

City:	State:	Zip:
Paynesville	TX	77777

Residence Phone:	County:	Social Security No.
999-976-9234	Broken Toe	675-97-9123

GUARANTOR

Name: SELF

Address:	RELN.	Guarantor No.
SAME		87333

City:	State:	Zip:

Phone:	Social Security:

EMPLOYER

Name: Data Base International

Address: 5675 International Blvd

City:	State:	Zip:
Duncanville	.TX	78666

Phone:	ADM By:	Occupation:
999-927-0347	C/M	COMPUTER ANALYST

Name:

Address:

City:	State:	Zip:

Phone:	Occupation:

INSURANCE

Insurance Company:	Plan #:	Group #:	Policy #:	Policy Holder:	Relation:	Sex:
TRAVELERS 4528 Medical Street SLC, UT 87433	67554	J09432	675-09876	Jack Daniels		

Admit Complaint:	Prvs. Admit This Hospital	Notify In Case Of Emergency:
chest pain/tightness	none	Jena Wade 987-009-7652

Comments: quadriplegia

NURSING ASSESMENT

Medications:

LTT	WT.		T	B/P	P	R
	145		98.6	133/82		

Physician: B. Mitchell

CONSENT TO TREATMENT: I, the undersigned hereby authorize St. Theresa Memorial Hospital to provide such medical care and to administer such laboratory procedures, radiological diagnostic and/or Therapeutic procedures and treatments, including but not limited to administration of pharmaceutical products, infusion or transfusion of blood or blood components, injections and intravenous medication or other therapeutic solutions as in the judgment of the physicians treating the patient may be deemed necessary and advisable. I understand I am entitled to have my own physician treat me, and he (she) will be called upon my request. I understand that a personal physician is to be selected by or on behalf of the patient within 24 hours if hospitalization or further treatment is required, or immediately if complaints arise. RELEASE OF INFORMATION: I hear-by authorize St. Theresa Memorial Hospital to release any information to any organization providing transportation to or from this hospital.

Signed: ____________________ Date: __________ Relationship to Patient ____________

If unable to sign, reason: ______________________________

Witness ______________ Witness ______________ Other Consent ______________

Physician Signature	Page No.	Title:
		Date:

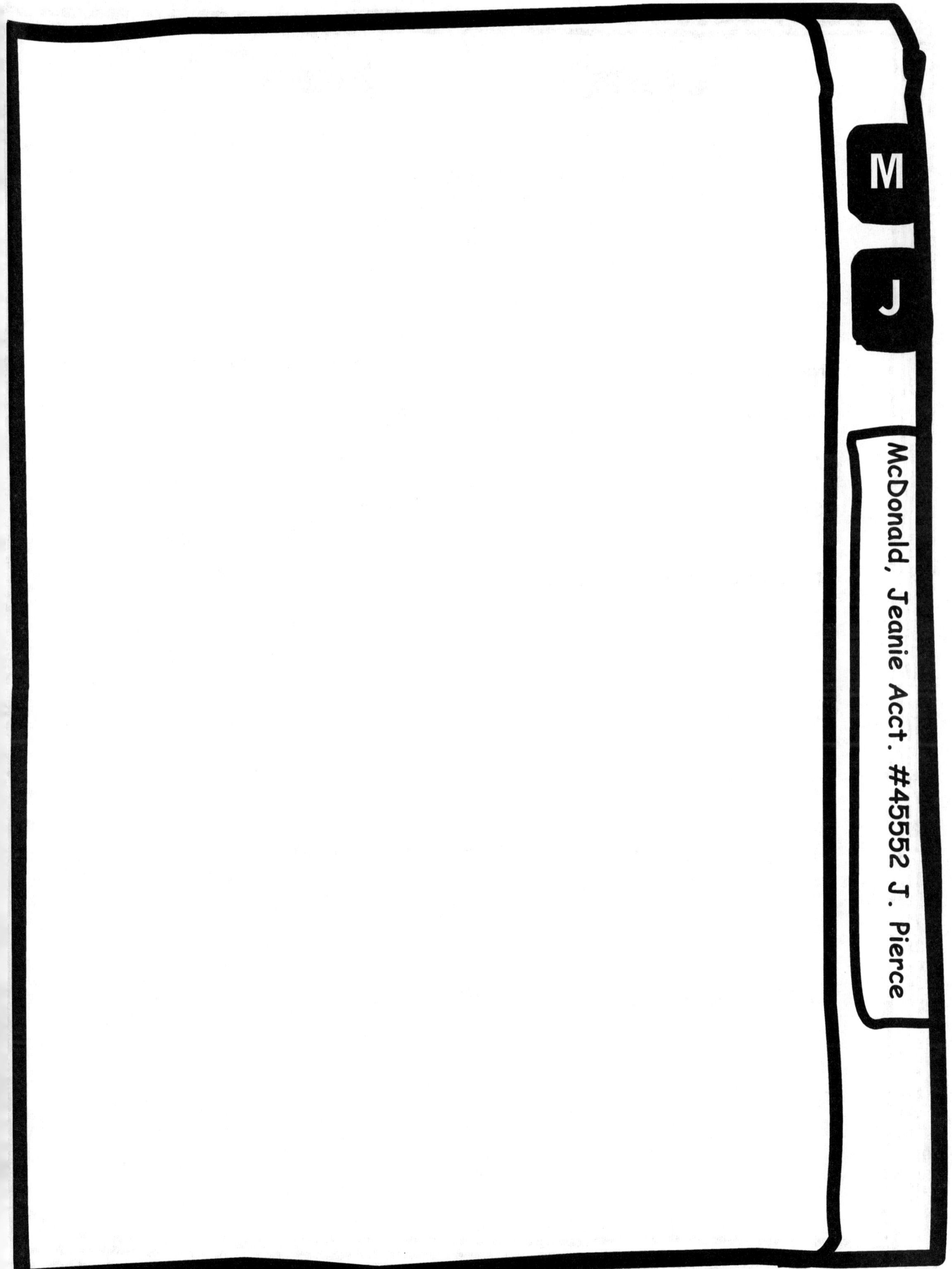
M
J
McDonald, Jeanie Acct. #45552 J. Pierce

Outpatient Services
St. Theresa's Hospital
Paynesville, Texas 77777

Name: Jeanie McDonald

Case #: R234810

Physician: J. Pierce

Date: 5/23/

Anesthetist:

Assistant:

Started:

Ended:

Diagnosis: Screening Mammogram. Last mammogram performed five years ago.

Operation:

Anesthesia:

INDICATIONS: 49 year-old admitted for Screening Mammogram

PROCEDURE: Screening Mammogram

OUTPATIENT RECORD

Account:	Physician:	Phy #:	Registration Date:	Time:	MSV:	Admit Category:	Med Rec. No.
45552	J. Pierce	JP2211	5/23	08:25		R	R234810

PATIENT

Name: Jeanie McDonald				
Address: 14333 Lakeside Drive	Religion: Jewish	DOB: 11/28	SEX: F	MS:
City: Paynesville	State: TX	Zip: 77777		
Residence Phone: 999-876-6655	County: Broken Toe	Social Security No. 787-44-1012		

EMPLOYER

Name: none		
Address:		
City:	State:	Zip:
Phone:	ADM By:	Occupation:

GUARANTOR

Name: Paul McDonald		
Address: same	RELN. Jewish	Guarantor No. P0097
City: Paynesville	State: TX	Zip: 77777
Phone: 999-876-2211	Social Security: 767-49-0099	

EMPLOYER

Name: Boardrooms Executive Offices		
Address: 101 West Buckingham Road		
City: Paynesville	State: TX	Zip: 77777
Phone: 999-757-8765	Occupation: office manager	

INSURANCE

Insurance Company:	Plan #:	Group #:	Policy #:	Policy Holder:	Relation:	Sex:
Martel Insurance Company 2451 Lake Street Lewsiville, OK 87654	H774	BEO99	12345	Paul McDonald	husband	M

Admit Complaint:	Prvs. Admit This Hospital	Notify In Case Of Emergency:
Screening mammogram	none	Paul McDonald

Comments:

NURSING ASSESMENT

Medications:
none

LTT	WT.		T	B/P	P	R
	156		99.8	120/80		

Physician:
J. Pierce

CONSENT TO TREATMENT: I, the undersigned hereby authorize St. Theresa Memorial Hospital to provide such medical care and to administer such laboratory procedures, radiological diagnostic and/or Therapeutic procedures and treatments, including but not limited to administration of pharmaceutical products, infusion or transfusion of blood or blood components, injections and intravenous medication or other therapeutic solutions as in the judgment of the physicians treating the patient may be deemed necessary and advisable. I understand I am entitled to have my own physician treat me, and he (she) will be called upon my request. I understand that a personal physician is to be selected by or on behalf of the patient within 24 hours if hospitalization or further treatment is required, or immediately if complaints arise. RELEASE OF INFORMATION: I hear-by authorize St. Theresa Memorial Hospital to release any information to any organization providing transportation to or from this hospital.

Signed: ______________________ Date: __________ Relationship to Patient ______________

If unable to sign, reason: ______________________________

Witness ______________ Witness ______________ Other Consent ______________

Physician Signature	Page No.	Title:
		Date:

M

J

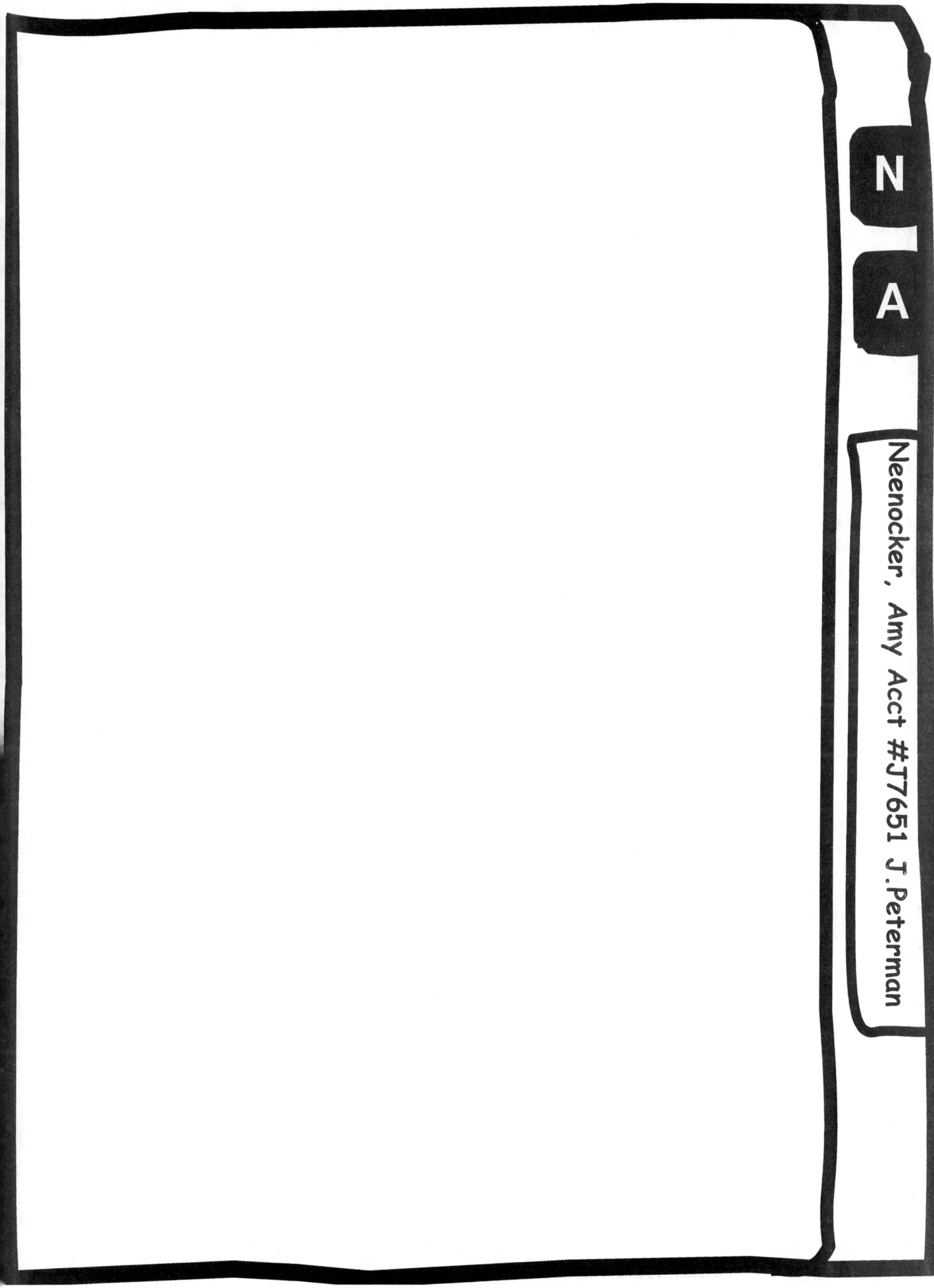
N
A
Neenocker, Amy Acct #J7651 J.Peterman

Outpatient Services

St. Theresa's Hospital
Paynesville, Texas 77777

Name: Amy Neenocker **Case #:** Q11707

Physician: J. Peterman **Date:** 3/18

Anesthetist: **Assistant:**

Started: **Ended:**

Preoperative Diagnosis: Recurrent Otitis Media
Tracheobronchial Malacia

Postoperative Diagnosis: Recurrent Otitis Media

Operation:

Anesthesia:

INDICATIONS: This 22-month old child has a history of severe Tracheobronchial Malacia requiring tracheotomy at 5 months of age as well as Gastrostomy tube placed at 5 months of age. Currently she has had recurrent ear infections and she is admitted for placement of tubes in her ears.

PROCEDURE: Bilateral Myringotomy with tube insertion

OUTPATIENT RECORD

Account:	Physician:	Phy #:	Registration Date:	Time:	MSV:	Admit Category:	Med Rec. No.
J7651	J. Peterman	JP0987	3/18	11:00			Q11707

PATIENT

Name:				
Amy Neenocker				
Address: 1542 Amberton Way	Religion: Presby.	DOB: 08/17	SEX: F	MS:
City: Paynesville	State: TX	Zip: 77777		
Residence Phone: 999-871-2929	County: Broken Toe	Social Security No. 765-09-0101		

GUARANTOR

Name: Paul and Amy Neenocker		
Address: SAME	RELN. SAME	Guarantor No. 7Y69876
City: SAME	State: SAME	Zip: SAME
Phone: SAME	Social Security: 964-09-1953	

EMPLOYER

Name:		
Address:		
City:	State:	Zip:
Phone:	ADM By: cm	Occupation:
Name:		
Address:		
City:	State:	Zip:
Phone:	Occupation:	

INSURANCE

Insurance Company:	Plan #:	Group #:	Policy #:	Policy Holder:	Relation:	Sex:
Kids Primary 9087 Alphabet Way New York, New York 87108	PK54	98176	G7109	Paul Neenocker	Father	M

Admit Complaint:	Prvs. Admit This Hospital	Notify In Case Of Emergency:
ears hurt	yes 11/23	parents see above

Comments:
history of tracheobronchial malacia and gastrostomy tube

NURSING ASSESMENT

Medications:
none

LTT	WT.		T	B/P	P	R
	25		99.9	145/95		

Physician:
J. Peterman

CONSENT TO TREATMENT: I, the undersigned hereby authorize St. Theresa Memorial Hospital to provide such medical care and to administer such laboratory procedures, radiological diagnostic and/or Therapeutic procedures and treatments, including but not limited to administration of pharmaceutical products, infusion or transfusion of blood or blood components, injections and intravenous medication or other therapeutic solutions as in the judgment of the physicians treating the patient may be deemed necessary and advisable. I understand I am entitled to have my own physician treat me, and he (she) will be called upon my request. I understand that a personal physician is to be selected by or on behalf of the patient within 24 hours if hospitalization or further treatment is required, or immediately if complaints arise. RELEASE OF INFORMATION: I hear-by authorize St. Theresa Memorial Hospital to release any information to any organization providing transportation to or from this hospital.

Signed: ____________________ Date: __________ Relationship to Patient ____________________

If unable to sign, reason: ____

Witness ____________________ Witness ____________________ Other Consent ____________________

Physician Signature	Page No.	Title:
		Date:

N

A

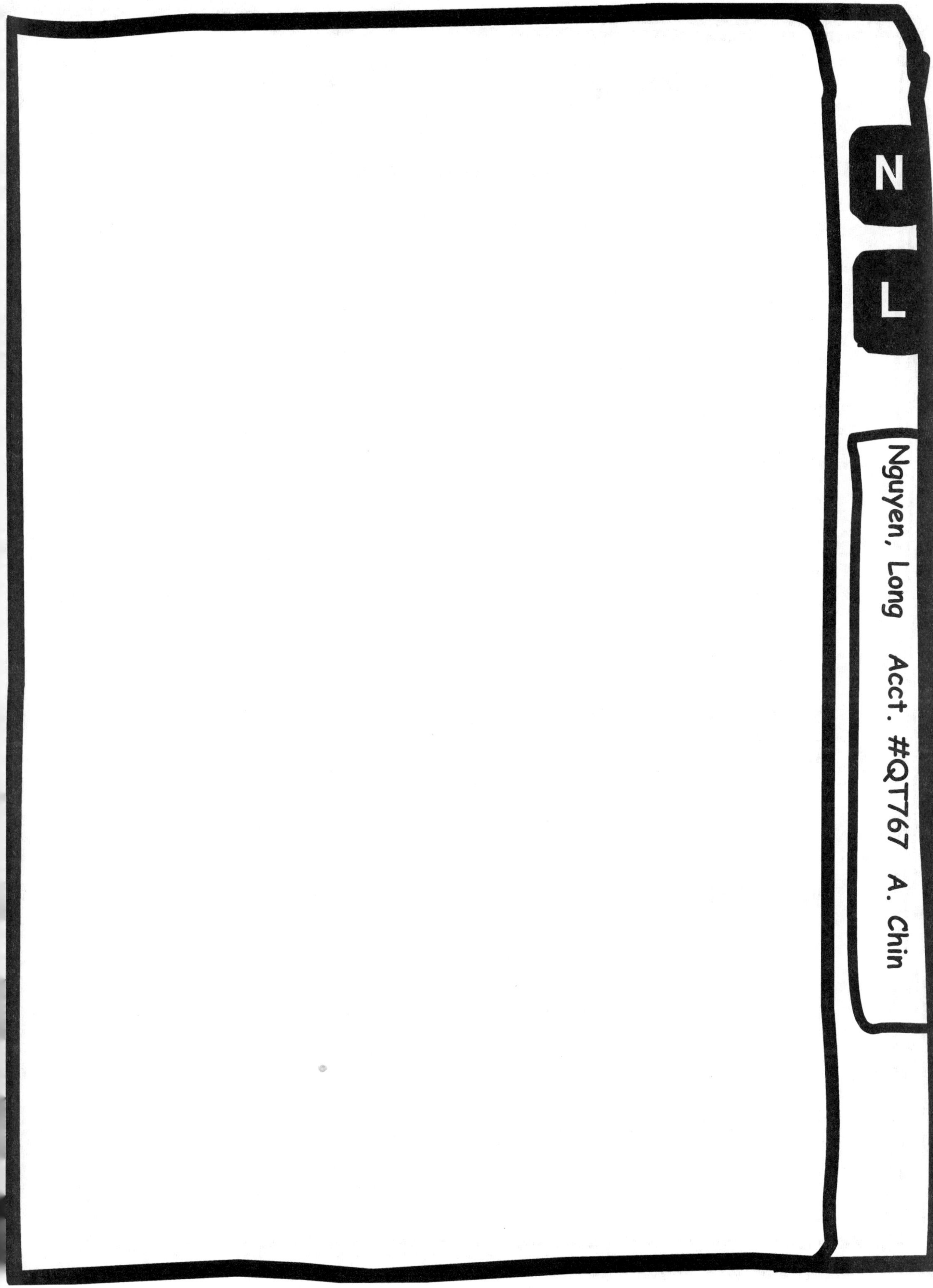
N
L
Nguyen, Long Acct. #QT767 A. Chin

Outpatient Services
St. Theresa's Hospital
Paynesville, Texas 77777

Name: Long Nguyen

Case #: O5683T

Physician: A. Chin

Date: 7/13/

Anesthetist:

Assistant:

Started:

Ended:

Diagnosis: Finger Injury; Knee Contusion; Head Contusion

INDICATIONS: 36 year-old admitted to the Emergency Room with multiple contusions. Double doors at local business hit patient. No fractures were visible on x-rays.

PROCEDURE: None.

OUTPATIENT RECORD

Account:	Physician:	Phy #:	Registration Date:	Time:	MSV:	Admit Category:	Med Rec. No.
QT767	A. Chin	AC776	7/13	09:00		ER	05683T

PATIENT

Name:				
Long Nguyen				
Address:	Religion	DOB:	SEX:	MS:
505 Hillcrest Lane #98	Buddist	09/16	M	
City:	State:	Zip:		
Paynesville	TX	77777		
Residence Phone:	County:	Social Security No.		
999-876-9292	Broken Toe	777-98-0099		

GUARANTOR

Name:		
self		
Address:	RELN.	Guarantor No.
City:	State:	Zip:
Phone:	Social Security:	

EMPLOYER

Name:			
Blue Band Broad Band			
Address:			
5413 Fast Way			
City:	State:	Zip:	
Paynesville	TX	77777	
Phone:	ADM By:	Occupation:	
999-876-0909			
Name:			
Address:			
City:	State:	Zip:	
Phone:	Occupation:		

INSURANCE

Insurance Company:	Plan #:	Group #:	Policy #:	Policy Holder:	Relation:	Sex:
Aetna Health 5432 Insurance Way Anytown, TX 87654	NB87	543-097	987656	Long Nguyen		M

Admit Complaint:	Prvs. Admit This Hospital	Notify In Case Of Emergency:
head pain	none	

Comments:
hit by doors

NURSING ASSESMENT

Medications:
none

LTT	WT.		T	B/P	P	R
	135		99.8	155/80		

Physician:
A. Chin

CONSENT TO TREATMENT: I, the undersigned hereby authorize St. Theresa Memorial Hospital to provide such medical care and to administer such laboratory procedures, radiological diagnostic and/or Therapeutic procedures and treatments, including but not limited to administration of pharmaceutical products, infusion or transfusion of blood or blood components, injections and intravenous medication or other therapeutic solutions as in the judgment of the physicians treating the patient may be deemed necessary and advisable. I understand I am entitled to have my own physician treat me, and he (she) will be called upon my request. I understand that a personal physician is to be selected by or on behalf of the patient within 24 hours if hospitalization or further treatment is required, or immediately if complaints arise. RELEASE OF INFORMATION: I hear-by authorize St. Theresa Memorial Hospital to release any information to any organization providing transportation to or from this hospital.

Signed: ______________________ Date: __________ Relationship to Patient______________

If unable to sign, reason: ______________________________________

Witness ____________________ Witness ____________________ Other Consent ______________

Physician Signature	Page No.	Title:
		Date:

N

L

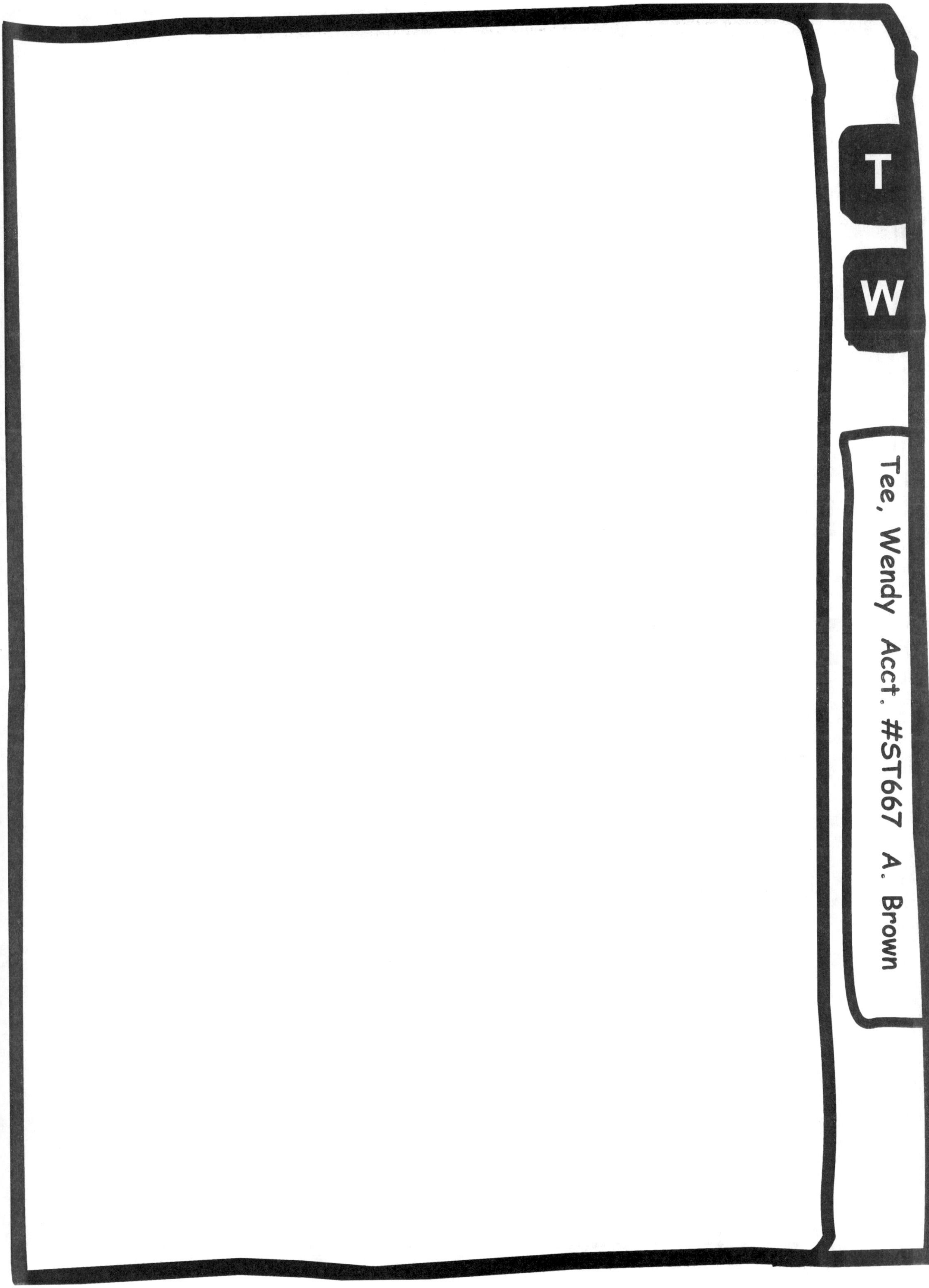
T
W
Tee, Wendy Acct. #ST667 A. Brown

Outpatient Services
St. Theresa's Hospital
Paynesville, Texas 77777

Name:	Wendy C. Tee	**Case #:**	A2384P
Physician:	A. Brown	**Date:**	4/19/
Anesthetist:		**Assistant:**	
Started:		**Ended:**	

Diagnosis: Epistaxis

INDICATIONS: 48 year-old admitted to the Emergency Room for Epistaxis. Patient has frequent nosebleeds. Also has Hypertension and Hypothyroidism. Nosebleed stopped with pressure and rest.

PROCEDURE:

OUTPATIENT RECORD

Account:	Physician:	Phy #:	Registration Date:	Time:	MSV:	Admit Category:	Med Rec. No.
ST667	A. Brown	B110	4/19	11:00		ER	A2384P

PATIENT

Name:				
Wendy C. Tee				
Address: 5510 Westin Heights	Religion: Baptist	DOB: 11/23	SEX: F	MS:
City: Paynesville	State: TX	Zip: 77777		
Residence Phone: 999-888-6565	County: Broken Toe	Social Security No. 555-66-7777		

GUARANTOR

Name:		
Mark Tee		
Address: same	RELN. none	Guarantor No. H88877
City: Paynesville	State: TX	Zip: 77777
Phone: 999-7776623	Social Security: 454-99-7777	

EMPLOYER

Name:		
Mullers Department Store		
Address: 1100 Ryan Street		
City: Paynesville	State: TX	Zip: 77777
Phone: 999-888-0909	ADM By: d/m	Occupation: clerk
Name: Whites		
Address: 7654 Preston Road		
City: Paynesville	State: TX	Zip: 77777
Phone: 999-434-7272	Occupation: manager	

INSURANCE

Insurance Company:	Plan #:	Group #:	Policy #:	Policy Holder:	Relation:	Sex:
BCBS 5525 Martel Lane Fort Smith, AR 66555	YH23	B5321	N33222	Mark Tee	husband	M

Admit Complaint:	Prvs. Admit This Hospital	Notify In Case Of Emergency:
nosebleed	none	Mark Tee see above

Comments:

NURSING ASSESMENT

Medications:
none

LTT	WT.		T	B/P	P	R
	95		99	165/95		

patient also has hypertension and hypothyroidism

Physician:
A. Brown

CONSENT TO TREATMENT: I, the undersigned hereby authorize St. Theresa Memorial Hospital to provide such medical care and to administer such laboratory procedures, radiological diagnostic and/or Therapeutic procedures and treatments, including but not limited to administration of pharmaceutical products, infusion or transfusion of blood or blood components, injections and intravenous medication or other therapeutic solutions as in the judgment of the physicians treating the patient may be deemed necessary and advisable. I understand I am entitled to have my own physician treat me, and he (she) will be called upon my request. I understand that a personal physician is to be selected by or on behalf of the patient within 24 hours if hospitalization or further treatment is required, or immediately if complaints arise. RELEASE OF INFORMATION: I hear-by authorize St. Theresa Memorial Hospital to release any information to any organization providing transportation to or from this hospital.

Signed: ______________________ Date: __________ Relationship to Patient______________

If unable to sign, reason: ______________________________

Witness ______________ Witness ______________ Other Consent ______________

Physician Signature	Page No.	Title: ER
	1	Date: 4/19

T

W

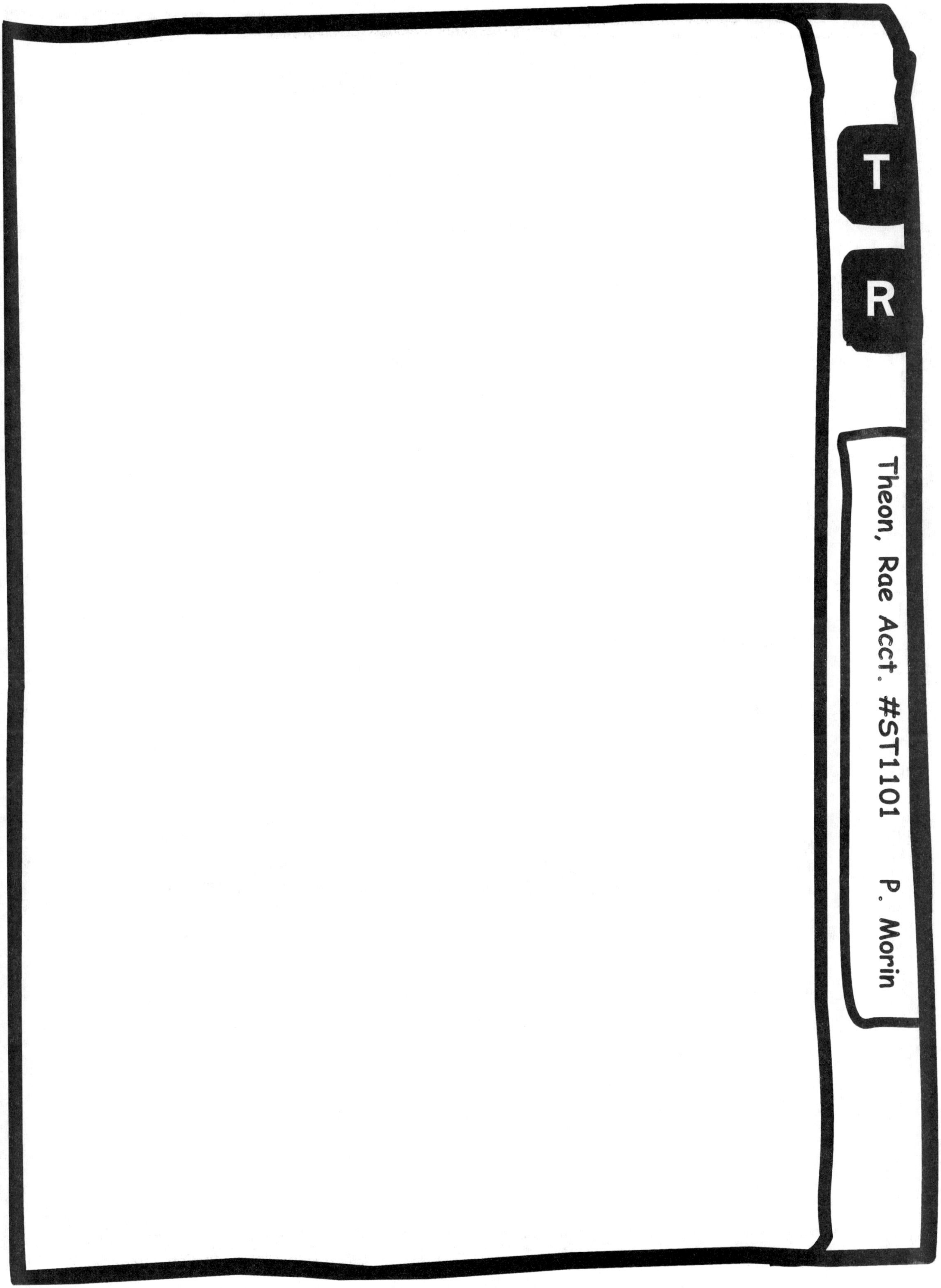
T
R
Theon, Rae Acct. #ST1101 P. Morin

Outpatient Services
St. Theresa's Hospital
Paynesville, Texas 77777

Name:	Rae Theon	**Case #:**	JJE508
Physician:	P. Morin	**Date:**	10-18
Anesthetist:	S. Pena	**Assistant:**	
Started:		**Ended:**	

Preoperative Diagnosis: Dysphagia, History of Proximal Esophageal Stricture

Postoperative Diagnosis: Proximal Esophageal Stricture Concentric

Operation:

Anesthesia:

INDICATIONS: 72 year old female with a history of proximal esophageal stricture of unclear etiology, possibly related to Fosamax, who has undergone repeat dilations, steriod injections and prolonged proton pump blocker therapy, with recurrent structuring.

PROCEDURE: Esophagogastroduodenoscopy with dilation of esophagus with balloons and injection of entralesional steroids.

OUTPATIENT RECORD

Account:	Physician:	Phy #:	Registration Date:	Time:	MSV:	Admit Category:	Med Rec. No.
ST1101	P. Morin	88150	10/18	07:00			JJE508

PATIENT

Name:				
Rae Theon				
Address: 101 Preston Road	Religion: Cath.	DOB: 10/22	SEX: F	MS:
City: Paynesville	State: TX	Zip: 77777		
Residence Phone: 999-555-1212	County: Broken Toe	Social Security No. 444-88-1111		

GUARANTOR

Name: Same		
Address:	RELN.	Guarantor No. 777-97-7777
City:	State:	Zip:
Phone:	Social Security:	

EMPLOYER

Name:		
Address:		
City:	State:	Zip:
Phone:	ADM By: d/m	Occupation:
Name:		
Address:		
City:	State:	Zip:
Phone:	Occupation:	

INSURANCE

Insurance Company:	Plan #:	Group #:	Policy #:	Policy Holder:	Relation:	Sex:
Blue Cross	A665	7610	BC1100	Rae Theon	self	F

Admit Complaint:	Prvs. Admit This Hospital	Notify In Case Of Emergency:
throat hurts	last year	Ben Albright 999-776-4920

Comments:
Has had problems in the past

NURSING ASSESMENT

Medications:
steroid injections
proton blocker therapy

LTT	WT.		T	B/P	P	R
	110		98.5	145/95		

Physician:
P. Morin

CONSENT TO TREATMENT: I, the undersigned hereby authorize St. Theresa Memorial Hospital to provide such medical care and to administer such laboratory procedures, radiological diagnostic and/or Therapeutic procedures and treatments, including but not limited to administration of pharmaceutical products, infusion or transfusion of blood or blood components, injections and intravenous medication or other therapeutic solutions as in the judgment of the physicians treating the patient may be deemed necessary and advisable. I understand I am entitled to have my own physician treat me, and he (she) will be called upon my request. I understand that a personal physician is to be selected by or on behalf of the patient within 24 hours if hospitalization or further treatment is required, or immediately if complaints arise. RELEASE OF INFORMATION: I hear-by authorize St. Theresa Memorial Hospital to release any information to any organization providing transportation to or from this hospital.

Signed: ______________________ Date: __________ Relationship to Patient ______________________

If unable to sign, reason: ____

Witness ______________________ Witness ______________________ Other Consent ______________________

Physician Signature	Page No.	Title: ER
	1	Date: 10/18

T

R

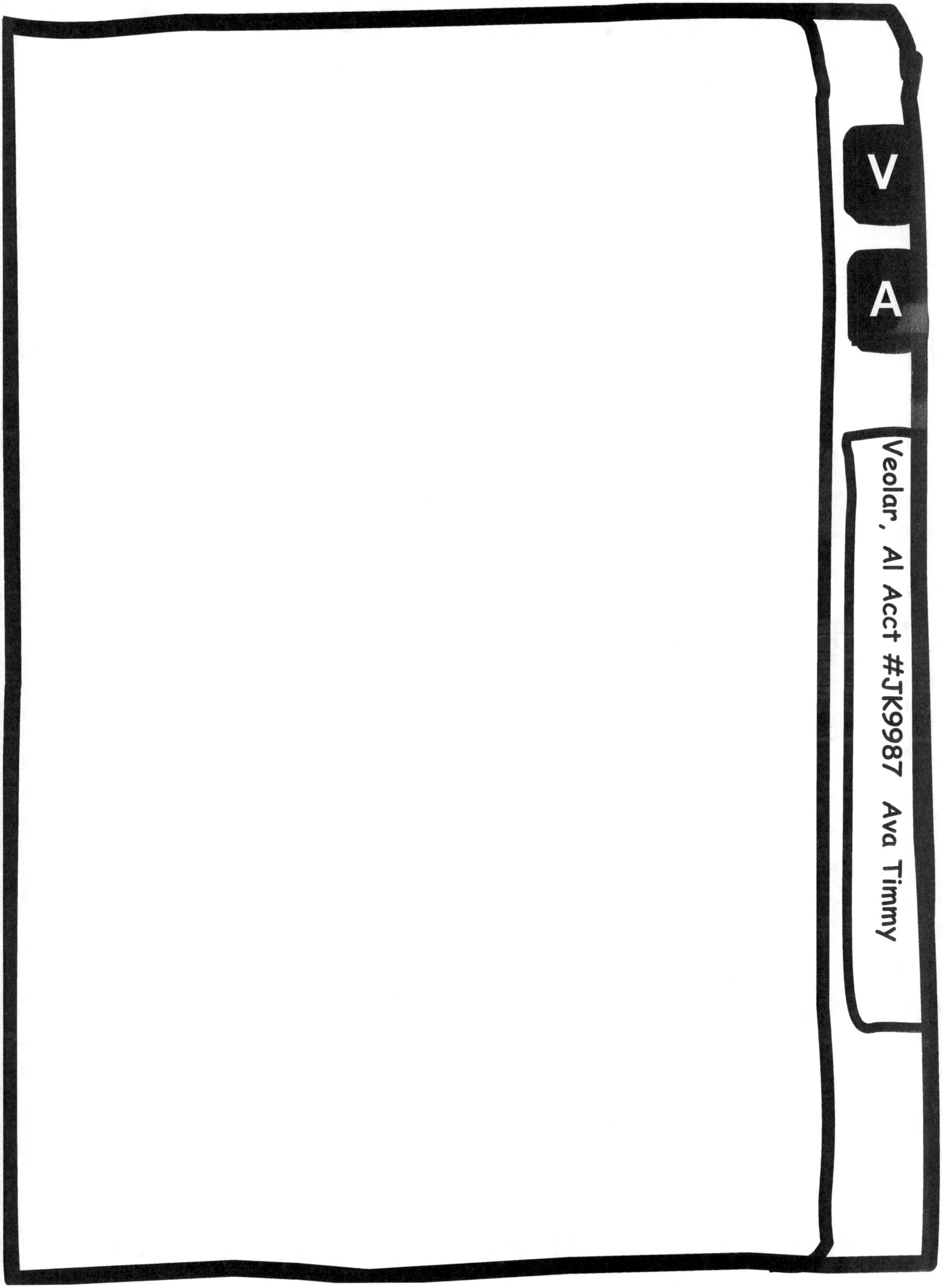
V
A
Veolar, Al Acct #JK9987 Ava Timmy

Outpatient Services
St. Theresa's Hospital
Paynesville, Texas 77777

Name:	Al Veolar	**Case #:**	J88210
Physician:	Ava Tummy	**Date:**	11/1/
Anesthetist:		**Assistant:**	
Started:		**Ended:**	

Preoperative Diagnosis: Displaced intra-articular fracture, base of right thumb

Postoperative Diagnosis: Displaced intra-articular fracture, base of right thumb

Operation:

Anesthesia:

INDICATIONS:

PROCEDURE: ORIF of right proximal phalanx thumb fracture

OUTPATIENT RECORD

Account:	Physician:	Phy #:	Registration Date:	Time:	MSV:	Admit Category:	Med Rec. No.
JK9987	Ava Tummy	AT9815	11/1	16:00		ER	J88210

PATIENT

Name:				
Al Veolar				
Address: 3567 Princeton	Religion	DOB: 03/24	SEX: M	MS:
City: Paynesville	State: TX	Zip: 77777		
Residence Phone: 999-898-0765	County: Broken Toe	Social Security No. 878-93-2752		

GUARANTOR

Name:		
SELF		
Address: SAME	RELN.	Guarantor No.
City:	State:	Zip:
Phone:	Social Security:	

EMPLOYER

Name:		
Wendells Plumbing		
Address: 7878 Latreen Street		
City: Paynesville	State: TX	Zip: 77777
Phone: 999-342-1234	ADM By: CM	Occupation: PLUMBER
Name:		
Address:		
City:	State:	Zip:
Phone:	Occupation:	

INSURANCE

Insurance Company:	Plan #:	Group #:	Policy #:	Policy Holder:	Relation:	Sex:
NONE						

Admit Complaint:	Prvs. Admit This Hospital	Notify In Case Of Emergency:
BROKEN FINGER	NONE	

Comments:

NURSING ASSESMENT

Medications:

LTT	WT.		T	B/P	P	R
	198		98.7	125/65		

Physician:
Ava Tummey

CONSENT TO TREATMENT: I, the undersigned hereby authorize St. Theresa Memorial Hospital to provide such medical care and to administer such laboratory procedures, radiological diagnostic and/or Therapeutic procedures and treatments, including but not limited to administration of pharmaceutical products, infusion or transfusion of blood or blood components, injections and intravenous medication or other therapeutic solutions as in the judgment of the physicians treating the patient may be deemed necessary and advisable. I understand I am entitled to have my own physician treat me, and he (she) will be called upon my request. I understand that a personal physician is to be selected by or on behalf of the patient within 24 hours if hospitalization or further treatment is required, or immediately if complaints arise. RELEASE OF INFORMATION: I hear-by authorize St. Theresa Memorial Hospital to release any information to any organization providing transportation to or from this hospital.

Signed: ______________________ Date: ___________ Relationship to Patient ______________________

If unable to sign, reason: ____

Witness ______________________ Witness ______________________ Other Consent ______________________

Physician Signature	Page No.	Title:
		Date:

V

A

	2.	3. PATIENT CONTROL NO.	4. TYPE OF BILL
	5. FED TAX NO.	6. STATEMENT COVERS PERIOD FROM / THROUGH	7. COV D
	8. N-O-D	9. C-I-D	10. L-A-D
	11.		
12. PATENT NAME	13. PATIENT ADDRESS		

14 D.O.B.	15 SEX	16 MS	17 DATE	18 HR	19 TYPE	20 SRO	21D HR	22 STAT	23 MEDICAL RECORD NO.	CONDITION CODES 24 / 26 / 28 / 30	31

32 OCCURANCE CODE	32 OCCURANCE DATE	34 OCCUR ANCE CODE	34 OCCUR ANCE DATE	36 OCCURANCE SPAN CODE	FROM	THROUGH	A B C	37

	39 VALUE CODES CODE	39 VALUE CODES AMOUNT	41 VALUE CODES CODE	41 VALUE CODES AMOUNT
a				
b				
c				
d				

42 REV CD	43 DESCRIPTION	44 HCPCS/RATES	45 SERV DATE	46 SERV UNITS	47 TOTAL CHARGES	48 NON-COVERED CHARGES	49

	50 PAYER	51 PROVIDER NO.	52 REL INFO	53 ASC NON	54 PAIOR PAYMENTS	55 EST AMOUNT DUE	56
A							
B							
C							
57		DUE FROM PATIENT					

58 INSURED'S NAME	59 P REL	60 CERT. - SSN-HIC.ID NO.	61 GROUP NAME	62 INSURNACE GROUP NO.	
					A
					B
					C

63 TREATMENT AUTHORIZATION CODES	64 ESC	65 EMPLOYER NAME	66 EMPLOYER LOCATION

67 PRIN DIAG CO	68 CODE (OTHER DIAG CODES)	70 CODE	72 CODE	74 CODE	76 ADMIN DIAG CD	77 E-CODE	78

67 P.C.	80 PRINCIPAL PRO CODE	80 PRINCIPAL PRO DATE	81 OTHER PROCEDURE CODE	81 OTHER PROCEDURE DATE	82 ATTENDING PHYS.ID	
						A
						B
	OTHER PROCEDURE CODE	OTHER PROCEDURE DATE	OTHER PROCEDURE CODE	OTHER PROCEDURE DATE	83 OTHER PHYS ID	A
						B
					OTHER PHYS ID	A
						B

84 REMARKS	85 PROVIDER REPRESENTIAVE	86 DATE
	X	

2. | 3. PATIENT CONTROL NO. | 4. TYPE OF BILL

5. FED TAX NO. | 6. STATEMENT COVERS PERIOD FROM THROUGH | 7. COV D | 8. N-O-D | 9. C-I-D | 10. L-A-D | 11.

12. PATENT NAME | 13. PATIENT ADDRESS

14 D.O.B. | 15 SEX | 16 MS | 17 DATE | 18 HR | 19 TYPE | 20 SRO | 21D HR | 22 STAT | 23 MEDICAL RECORD NO. | CONDITION CODES 24 26 28 30 | 31

32 OCCURANCE CODE DATE | 34 OCCUR ANCE CODE DATE | 36 OCCURANCE SPAN CODE FROM THROUGH | A B C | 37

a b c d | 39 VALUE CODES CODE AMOUNT | 41VALUE CODES CODE AMOUNT

42 REV CD | 43 DESCRIPTION | 44 HCPCS/RATES | 45 SERV DATE | 46 SERV UNITS | 47 TOTAL CHARGES | 48 NON-COVERED CHARGES | 49

1 2 3 4 5 6 7 8 9 0 1 2 3 4 5 6 7 8 9 0 1 2 3

50 PAYER | 51 PROVIDER NO. | 52REL INFO | 53 ASC NON | 54 PAIOR PAYMENTS | 55 EST AMOUNT DUE | 56

A B C

57 | DUE FROM PATIENT

58 INSURED'S NAME | 59 P REL | 60 CERT. - SSN-HIC.ID NO. | 61 GROUP NAME | 62 INSURNACE GROUP NO. | A B C

63 TREATMENT AUTHORIZATION CODES | 64 ESC | 65 EMPLOYER NAME | 66 EMPLOYER LOCATION

67 PRIN DIAG CO | OTHER DIAG CODES 68 CODE 70 CODE 72 CODE 74 CODE | 76 ADMIN DIAG CD | 77 E-CODE | 78

67 P.C. | 80 PRINCIPAL PRO CODE DATE | 81 OTHER PROCEDURE CODE DATE | 82 ATTENDING PHYS.ID A B

OTHER PROCEDURE CODE DATE | OTHER PROCEDURE CODE DATE | 83 OTHER PHYS ID A B | OTHER PHYS ID A B

84 REMARKS | 85 PROVIDER REPRESENTIAVE | 86 DATE

X

2.

3. PATIENT CONTROL NO.

4. TYPE OF BILL

5. FED TAX NO. | 6. STATEMENT COVERS PERIOD FROM THROUGH | 7. COV D | 8. N-O-D | 9. C-I-D | 10. L-A-D | 11.

12. PATENT NAME | 13. PATIENT ADDRESS

14 D.O.B. | 15 SEX | 16 MS | 17 DATE | 18 HR | 19 TYPE | 20 SRO | 21D HR | 22 STAT | 23 MEDICAL RECORD NO. | CONDITION CODES 24 26 28 30 | 31

32 OCCURANCE CODE DATE | 34 OCCUR ANCE CODE DATE | 36 OCCURANCE SPAN CODE FROM THROUGH | A B C | 37

a b c d | 39 VALUE CODES CODE AMOUNT | 41VALUE CODES CODE AMOUNT

42 REV CD	43 DESCRIPTION	44 HCPCS/RATES	45 SERV DATE	46 SERV UNITS	47 TOTAL CHARGES	48 NON-COVERED CHARGES	49

1 2 3 4 5 6 7 8 9 0 1 2 3 4 5 6 7 8 9 0 1 2 3

50 PAYER | 51 PROVIDER NO. | 52REL INFO | 53 ASC NON | 54 PAIOR PAYMENTS | 55 EST AMOUNT DUE | 56

A B C

57 DUE FROM PATIENT

58 INSURED'S NAME | 59 P REL | 60 CERT. - SSN-HIC.ID NO. | 61 GROUP NAME | 62 INSURNACE GROUP NO. | A B C

63 TREATMENT AUTHORIZATION CODES | 64 ESC | 65 EMPLOYER NAME | 66 EMPLOYER LOCATION

67 PRIN DIAG CO | OTHER DIAG CODES 68 CODE 70 CODE 72 CODE 74 CODE | 76 ADMIN DIAG CD | 77 E-CODE | 78

67 P.C. | 80 PRINCIPAL PRO CODE DATE | 81 OTHER PROCEDURE CODE DATE

82 ATTENDING PHYS.ID A B

OTHER PROCEDURE CODE DATE | OTHER PROCEDURE CODE DATE

83 OTHER PHYS ID A B

OTHER PHYS ID A B

84 REMARKS

85 PROVIDER REPRESENTIAVE | 86 DATE

X

	2.		3. PATIENT CONTROL NO.	4. TYPE OF BILL

5. FED TAX NO.	6. STATEMENT COVERS PERIOD FROM	THROUGH	7. COV D	8. N-O-D	9. C-I-D	10. L-A-D	11.

12. PATENT NAME	13. PATIENT ADDRESS

14 D.O.B.	15 SEX	16 MS	17 DATE	18 HR	19 TYPE	20 SRO	21D HR	22 STAT	23 MEDICAL RECORD NO.	CONDITION CODES 24	26	28	30	31

32 OCCURANCE		34 OCCUR ANCE		36 OCCURANCE SPAN			A B C	37
CODE	DATE	CODE	DATE	CODE	FROM	THROUGH		

	39 VALUE CODES		41VALUE CODES	
	CODE	AMOUNT	CODE	AMOUNT
a				
b				
c				
d				

	42 REV CD	43 DESCRIPTION	44 HCPCS/RATES	45 SERV DATE	46 SERV UNITS	47 TOTAL CHARGES	48 NON-COVERED CHARGES	49	
1									1
2									2
3									3
4									4
5									5
6									6
7									7
8									8
9									9
0									0
1									1
2									2
3									3
4									4
5									5
6									6
7									7
8									8
9									9
0									0
1									1
2									2
3									3

	50 PAYER	51 PROVIDER NO.	52REL INFO	53 ASC NON	54 PAIOR PAYMENTS	55 EST AMOUNT DUE	56
A							
B							
C							

57 DUE FROM PATIENT

58 INSURED'S NAME	59 P REL	60 CERT. - SSN-HIC.ID NO.	61 GROUP NAME	62 INSURNACE GROUP NO.	
					A
					B
					C

63 TREATMENT AUTHORIZATION CODES	64 ESC	65 EMPLOYER NAME	66 EMPLOYER LOCATION

67 PRIN DIAG CO	OTHER DIAG CODES 68 CODE	70 CODE	72 CODE	74 CODE	76 ADMIN DIAG CD	77 E-CODE	78

67 P.C.	80 PRINCIPAL PRO		81 OTHER PROCEDURE	
	CODE	DATE	CODE	DATE

OTHER PROCEDURE		OTHER PROCEDURE	
CODE	DATE	CODE	DATE

82 ATTENDING PHYS.ID	A
	B
83 OTHER PHYS ID	A
	B
OTHER PHYS ID	A
	B

84 REMARKS

85 PROVIDER REPRESENTIAVE | 86 DATE

X

2.	3. PATIENT CONTROL NO.	4. TYPE OF BILL

5. FED TAX NO.	6. STATEMENT COVERS PERIOD FROM	THROUGH	7. COV D	8. N-O-D	9. C-I-D	10. L-A-D	11.

12. PATENT NAME	13. PATIENT ADDRESS

14 D.O.B.	15 SEX	16 MS	17 DATE	18 HR	19 TYPE	20 SRO	21D HR	22 STAT	23 MEDICAL RECORD NO.	CONDITION CODES 24	25	26	27	28	29	30	31

32 OCCURANCE CODE	DATE		34 OCCUR ANCE CODE	DATE		36 OCCURANCE SPAN CODE	FROM	THROUGH	A B C	37

	a b c d	39 VALUE CODES CODE	AMOUNT			41VALUE CODES CODE	AMOUNT

	42 REV CD	43 DESCRIPTION	44 HCPCS/RATES	45 SERV DATE	46 SERV UNITS	47 TOTAL CHARGES	48 NON-COVERED CHARGES	49	
1									1
2									2
3									3
4									4
5									5
6									6
7									7
8									8
9									9
0									0
1									1
2									2
3									3
4									4
5									5
6									6
7									7
8									8
9									9
0									0
1									1
2									2
3									3

	50 PAYER	51 PROVIDER NO.	52REL INFO	53 ASC NON	54 PAIOR PAYMENTS	55 EST AMOUNT DUE	56
A							
B							
C							
57		DUE FROM PATIENT					

58 INSURED'S NAME	59 P REL	60 CERT. - SSN-HIC.ID NO.	61 GROUP NAME	62 INSURNACE GROUP NO.	
					A B C

63 TREATMENT AUTHORIZATION CODES	64 ESC	65 EMPLOYER NAME	66 EMPLOYER LOCATION

67 PRIN DIAG CO	OTHER DIAG CODES 68 CODE		70 CODE		72 CODE		74 CODE		76 ADMIN DIAG CD	77 E-CODE	78

67 P.C.	80 PRINCIPAL PRO CODE	DATE	81 OTHER PROCEDURE CODE	DATE		82 ATTENDING PHYS.ID	A
							B
	OTHER PROCEDURE CODE	DATE		OTHER PROCEDURE CODE	DATE	83 OTHER PHYS ID	A
							B
						OTHER PHYS ID	A
							B

84 REMARKS	85 PROVIDER REPRESENTIAVE	86 DATE
	X	

	2.	3. PATIENT CONTROL NO.	4. TYPE OF BILL

5. FED TAX NO.	6. STATEMENT COVERS PERIOD FROM	THROUGH	7. COV D	8. N-O-D	9. C-I-D	10. L-A-D	11.

12. PATENT NAME	13. PATIENT ADDRESS

14 D.O.B.	15 SEX	16 MS	17 DATE	18 HR	19 TYPE	20 SRO	21D HR	22 STAT	23 MEDICAL RECORD NO.	CONDITION CODES 24	26	28	30	31

32 OCCURANCE CODE	DATE	34 OCCUR ANCE CODE	DATE	36 OCCURANCE SPAN CODE	FROM	THROUGH	A B C	37

	39 VALUE CODES CODE	AMOUNT	41VALUE CODES CODE	AMOUNT
a				
b				
c				
d				

	42 REV CD	43 DESCRIPTION	44 HCPCS/RATES	45 SERV DATE	46 SERV UNITS	47 TOTAL CHARGES	48 NON-COVERED CHARGES	49	
1									1
2									2
3									3
4									4
5									5
6									6
7									7
8									8
9									9
0									0
1									1
2									2
3									3
4									4
5									5
6									6
7									7
8									8
9									9
0									0
1									1
2									2
3									3

	50 PAYER	51 PROVIDER NO.	52REL INFO	53 ASC NON	54 PAIOR PAYMENTS	55 EST AMOUNT DUE	56
A							
B							
C							
57		DUE FROM PATIENT					

58 INSURED'S NAME	59 P REL	60 CERT. - SSN-HIC.ID NO.	61 GROUP NAME	62 INSURNACE GROUP NO.	
					A
					B
					C

63 TREATMENT AUTHORIZATION CODES	64 ESC	65 EMPLOYER NAME	66 EMPLOYER LOCATION

67 PRIN DIAG CO	OTHER DIAG CODES 68 CODE	70 CODE	72 CODE	74 CODE	76 ADMIN DIAG CD	77 E-CODE	78

67 P.C.	80 PRINCIPAL PRO CODE	DATE	81 OTHER PROCEDURE CODE	DATE
	OTHER PROCEDURE CODE	DATE	OTHER PROCEDURE CODE	DATE

82 ATTENDING PHYS.ID	A
	B
83 OTHER PHYS ID	A
	B
OTHER PHYS ID	A
	B

84 REMARKS

85 PROVIDER REPRESENTIAVE	86 DATE
X	

	2.	3. PATIENT CONTROL NO.	4. TYPE OF BILL

5. FED TAX NO.	6. STATEMENT COVERS PERIOD FROM	THROUGH	7. COV D	8. N-O-D	9. C-I-D	10. L-A-D	11.

12. PATENT NAME	13. PATIENT ADDRESS

14 D.O.B.	15 SEX	16 MS	17 DATE	18 HR	19 TYPE	20 SRO	21D HR	22 STAT	23 MEDICAL RECORD NO.	CONDITION CODES 24	26	28	30	31

32 OCCURANCE		34 OCCUR ANCE		36 OCCURANCE SPAN			A B C	37
CODE	DATE	CODE	DATE	CODE	FROM	THROUGH		

	39 VALUE CODES		41VALUE CODES	
	CODE	AMOUNT	CODE	AMOUNT
a				
b				
c				
d				

42 REV CD	43 DESCRIPTION	44 HCPCS/RATES	45 SERV DATE	46 SERV UNITS	47 TOTAL CHARGES	48 NON-COVERED CHARGES	49
1							1
2							2
3							3
4							4
5							5
6							6
7							7
8							8
9							9
0							0
1							1
2							2
3							3
4							4
5							5
6							6
7							7
8							8
9							9
0							0
1							1
2							2
3							3

	50 PAYER	51 PROVIDER NO.	52REL INFO	53 ASC NON	54 PAIOR PAYMENTS	55 EST AMOUNT DUE	56
A							
B							
C							

57 DUE FROM PATIENT

58 INSURED'S NAME	59 P REL	60 CERT. - SSN-HIC.ID NO.	61 GROUP NAME	62 INSURNACE GROUP NO.	A B C

63 TREATMENT AUTHORIZATION CODES	64 ESC	65 EMPLOYER NAME	66 EMPLOYER LOCATION

67 PRIN DIAG CO	OTHER DIAG CODES 68 CODE	70 CODE	72 CODE	74 CODE	76 ADMIN DIAG CD	77 E-CODE	78

67 P.C.	80 PRINCIPAL PRO		81 OTHER PROCEDURE	
	CODE	DATE	CODE	DATE

OTHER PROCEDURE		OTHER PROCEDURE	
CODE	DATE	CODE	DATE

82 ATTENDING PHYS.ID	A
	B
83 OTHER PHYS ID	A
	B
OTHER PHYS ID	A
	B

84 REMARKS

85 PROVIDER REPRESENTIAVE 86 DATE

X

	2.	3. PATIENT CONTROL NO.	4. TYPE OF BILL

5. FED TAX NO.	6. STATEMENT COVERS PERIOD FROM	THROUGH	7. COV D	8. N-O-D	9. C-I-D	10. L-A-D	11.

12. PATENT NAME	13. PATIENT ADDRESS

14 D.O.B.	15 SEX	16 MS	17 DATE	18 HR	19 TYPE	20 SRO	21D HR	22 STAT	23 MEDICAL RECORD NO.	CONDITION CODES 24	26	28	30	31

32 OCCURANCE CODE	DATE	34 OCCUR ANCE CODE	DATE	36 OCCURANCE SPAN CODE	FROM	THROUGH	A B C	37

	39 VALUE CODES CODE	AMOUNT		41VALUE CODES CODE	AMOUNT
a					
b					
c					
d					

	42 REV CD	43 DESCRIPTION	44 HCPCS/RATES	45 SERV DATE	46 SERV UNITS	47 TOTAL CHARGES	48 NON-COVERED CHARGES	49	
1									1
2									2
3									3
4									4
5									5
6									6
7									7
8									8
9									9
0									0
1									1
2									2
3									3
4									4
5									5
6									6
7									7
8									8
9									9
0									0
1									1
2									2
3									3

	50 PAYER	51 PROVIDER NO.	52REL INFO	53 ASC NON	54 PAIOR PAYMENTS	55 EST AMOUNT DUE	56
A							
B							
C							
57		DUE FROM PATIENT					

58 INSURED'S NAME	59 P REL	60 CERT. - SSN-HIC.ID NO.	61 GROUP NAME	62 INSURNACE GROUP NO.	
					A
					B
					C

63 TREATMENT AUTHORIZATION CODES	64 ESC	65 EMPLOYER NAME	66 EMPLOYER LOCATION

67 PRIN DIAG CO	OTHER DIAG CODES 68 CODE	70 CODE	72 CODE	74 CODE	76 ADMIN DIAG CD	77 E-CODE	78

67 P.C.	80 PRINCIPAL PRO CODE	DATE	81 OTHER PROCEDURE CODE	DATE

OTHER PROCEDURE CODE	DATE	OTHER PROCEDURE CODE	DATE

82 ATTENDING PHYS.ID	A
	B
83 OTHER PHYS ID	A
	B
OTHER PHYS ID	A
	B

84 REMARKS

85 PROVIDER REPRESENTIAVE	86 DATE
X	

MedBooks Order Form

1-800-443-7397

Date:__________

Company Name:______________________________

Company Contact:______________________________

Telephone Number:______________ Fax Number:______________

UPS Address:______________________________

____

______________________________ Email Address:______________

Quantity	Description	Unit Price	Total Price
______	CP"Teach" Textbook	44.95	______
______	CP"Teach" Student Workbook	29.95	______
______	CP"Teach" Student Workbook w/Answers	34.95	______
______	Advanced Case Study Workbook	34.95	______
______	CP"Teach" Instructor's Manual	199.95	______
______	Instructor's Manual Refill	69.95	______
The above CP"Teach" titles offer a 20% discount for orders of 11+ on individual titles			
______	CPT Manual (Softbound)	49.95	______
______	CPT Manual (Spiralbound)	54.95	______
______	CPT Manual (other formats/call for pricing)		______
______	HCPCS National Codes	49.95	______
______	ICD-9-CM Easy Coder	59.95	______
______	ICD-9 Color Coded, Vols. 1, 2, 3 (Professional)	79.95	______
______	ICD-9 Color Coded, Vols. 1 & 2	53.95	______
______	RBRVS	71.95	______
______	Other (call for pricing)		

Call for SHIPPING ______

SUBTOTAL ______

8.25% Sales Tax (Texas Residents Only) ______

TOTAL $______

____ VISA ____ MasterCard ____ Am Express ____ Check (payable to MedBooks)

Card Number ______________________________ Expiration Date _____/_____

Cardholder's Name ______________________________ (please print)

Thank You for Choosing MedBooks! Call for information on Coding Seminars!

Please fax order to 972-994-0215